Young People, Class and Place

Under the weight of apparently growing consumer affluence, globalisation and post-modern social theory, many have proclaimed the declining significance of social class and place to young people's lives – and for social science. Drawing upon new, empirically grounded, theoretically innovative studies, this volume begs to differ.

It argues that the youth phase provides a privileged vantage point from which to interrogate and think about broader processes of social change and social continuity. These themes are addressed by all the diverse contributions gathered here. The chapters include investigation of: the problems of growing up in gang neighbourhoods and young people's use of space for leisure; new patterns of class formation and youth transition in Eastern Europe; the effects of classed labels and identities (such as 'chav' and 'charver') in youth culture and schooling; the changing meanings of class and place for young women in changing socio-economic landscapes; new patterns of youth culture and transition among Black young men in East London; and how we think and theorise about change and continuity in youth studies.

Together these new empirical studies and critical theoretical analyses confirm the continuing importance of class and place in shaping the opportunities, transitions, sub-cultures and life-styles of young people.

This book was based on a special issue of *Journal of Youth Studies.*

Robert MacDonald is Professor of Sociology at Teesside University.

Tracy Shildrick is Reader in Sociology at Teesside University.

Shane Blackman is Reader in Sociology and Cultural Studies at Canterbury Christ Church University.

Young People, Class and Place

Edited by Robert MacDonald, Tracy Shildrick
and Shane Blackman

Routledge
Taylor & Francis Group
LONDON AND NEW YORK

First published 2010 by Routledge
2 Park Square, Milton Park, Abingdon, Oxon, OX14 4RN

Simultaneously published in the USA and Canada
by Routledge
270 Madison Avenue, New York, NY 10016

Routledge is an imprint of the Taylor & Francis Group, an informa business

This book is a reproduction of the *Journal of Youth Studies*, vol. 12, issue 5. The Publisher requests to those authors who may be citing this book to state, also, the bibliographical details of the special issue on which the book was based

Typeset in Times by Value Chain, India
Printed and bound in Great Britain by TJI Digital, Padstow, Cornwall

British Library Cataloguing in Publication Data
A catalogue record for this book is available from the British Library

ISBN10: 0-415-56756-4
ISBN13: 978-0-415-56756-5

CONTENTS

1	Young people, class and place *Tracy Shildrick, Shane Blackman and Robert MacDonald*	1
2	Constructions of the working-class 'Other' among urban, white, middle-class youth: 'chavs', subculture and the valuing of education *Sumi Hollingworth and Katya Williams*	10
3	Who needs enemies with friends like these? The importance of place for young people living in known gang areas *Robert Ralphs, Juanjo Medina and Judith Aldridge*	26
4	'Nightscapes and leisure spaces': an ethnographic study of young people's use of free space *Cara Robinson*	44
5	Grafting, going to college and working on road: youth transitions and cultures in an East London neighbourhood *Anthony Gunter and Paul Watt*	58
6	From 'inheritance' to individualization: disembedding working-class youth transitions in post-Soviet Russia *Charlie Walker*	73
7	Steps and stages: rethinking transitions in youth and place *Tom Hall, Amanda Coffey and Brett Lashua*	88
8	(Re)constituting the past, (re)branding the present and (re)imagining the future: women's spatial negotiation of gender and class *Yvette Taylor and Michelle Addison*	103
9	New class divisions in the new market economies: evidence from the careers of young adults in post-Soviet Armenia, Azerbaijan and Georgia *Ken Roberts and Gary Pollock*	119
	Index	137

Young people, class and place

Tracy Shildrick[a], Shane Blackman[b] and Robert MacDonald[a]

[a]*Youth Research Group, School of Social Sciences and Law, University of Teesside, Middlesbrough, UK;* [b]*Department of Media, Canterbury Christ Church University, Canterbury, UK*

This collection focuses on issues of class and place in respect of young people's lives. The contributions derive, at least in part, from a one-day British Sociological Association Youth Study Group seminar that was hosted by the Youth Research Group at the University of Teesside in September 2008. We were overwhelmed with proposals to present papers – and a little surprised, given the supposed declining power of 'old' social divisions to explain contemporary society.

We might ask, what is special or important about the social scientific study of youth? One answer is that the youth phase provides a privileged vantage point from which to observe broader processes of social change and social continuity (Furlong and Cartmel 2007, MacDonald and Shildrick 2009). If new cultural trends emerge or significant social developments happen, it is feasible that they will be seen here first or most obviously, among the coming, new generation of young adults. If 'choice biographies' replace 'normal' ones, if family or household forms become less standard, if well-known patterns of gender or class inequality loosen or become less familiar, it is likely that these changes will be observed first in youth; changes made by young people as they make transitions to adult life. And while other life phases also involve transitions, transitions in youth – from childhood to adulthood – are, to us, the most significant. This is regardless of metaphors other than 'transition' that we might prefer, the blurring of age categories, and the nature of youth transitions (e.g. whether they be extended, fragmented, 'broken' or not). Andy Furlong and Fred Cartmel (2007, p. 2) make the same point: 'The study of youth provides an ideal opportunity to examine the relevance of new social theories; if the social order has changed and if social structures have weakened, we would expect to find evidence of these changes among young people who are at the crossroads of social reproduction.'

Our aim in hosting the seminar, and in producing this volume, was to encourage new, empirically grounded, theoretically informed discussions of either social class or place in the lives of young people in the current period. We are very grateful to the authors for fulfilling this aim. Their papers point to the value of an interdisciplinary perspective on young lives and draw upon sociology, cultural studies, criminology, urban studies, architecture, town planning, urban regeneration, and geography. The special edition illustrates the importance of both cultural and material aspects of class and place, and, more or less prominently, all the authors confront questions of social change and continuity, drawing on first-hand research with young people in a diversity of social situations and geographic locations.

The class question

Social class for a period became rather unfashionable even if some researchers have remained steadfast in their analyses of the pervasive effects of social class processes (Byrne 2005, Skeggs 2005). In our collection we find a renewed focus on social class relations as a source of both contestation and solidarity. The volume demonstrates the modern legacy of Karl Marx's idea that social class continues to be a divisive element of today's social structure. For Marx, social classes experience constant challenge under 'new conditions of oppression . . . and new forms of struggle in place of the old ones'.[1] He understood that forces of global, corporate capital shape social class formation, stating: 'The bourgeoisie has through its exploitation of the world market given a cosmopolitan character to production and consumption in every country.' Marx was aware of how the social relations of consumption and production change. For him, capital 'is a social power' and through young people's passion for brands, products and labels, we see how they are attracted towards what Marx (1887, pp. 76–81) called the magical capacity of the commodity to transform our identities. In these different papers we see young people under pressure to gain employment and education, striving for identity, and engaging in legal and illegal activities as they struggle with restricted job opportunities. In 2010, under new economic conditions of recession, we see many young people experiencing contradictions of high expectation and low outcome. Youth culture is surrounded by international and cosmopolitan images, which speak of dynamism and opportunity, but these seductions of globalization can appear fluid or elusive without material resources. As Skeggs *et al.* (2008, p. 6) point out, 'self-reflexivity does not offer the uncoupling of agency from structure'; rather, 'self-reflexivity itself depends upon access to resources and concomitant forms of capital.' Lack of resources in itself does not prevent active and reflexive choice and decision-making, but it surely serves to limit the options for such, in some cases severely. Young people want the products of global corporate companies like McDonalds, Nike and Coca-Cola; these images speak of youth having pleasure within an international setting free of the tyranny of locality.

David Harvey (2005, p. 149) describes this process as 'accumulation by dispossession' whereby the corporate companies, for example, through sponsorship take away the resources and culture of people at the level of the local. This contradiction is captured by Fredric Jameson's (2000) analysis of the power of generalized corporate culture, which can harness the seductions of advertisements and consumption, and promote itself as liberating for all individuals, thereby removing the need for location and place as these become identified as forms of oppression derived from local space which in turn holds people back, acting as a form of constraint. From a critical position, Manuel Castells (1989) sees these actions as the annihilation of space; here young people are either excluded from spaces or subject to surveillance in their own place, thereby making it seem that youth want to destroy where they live through graffiti and vandalism, but at the same time through some of these actions young people speak of the importance and identity of their location. Either way, young people are faced with the irony that under globalization place is becoming more important as they experience an increased priority of the specificity of locality. Social policies based on the principle of social exclusion, ostracize youth from their own space, making it appear that the only place that government sanctions for young people is their home. Thus, young people face mounting tensions and surveillance at home, on the street or in the park as they seek to capture what adults already possess, their own place.

Theoretical questions about class (less so about place) have been to the fore within Anglophone youth studies in recent years. Key has been the extent to which the old and prime social division of modernity, by social class, still 'works' in explaining the lives of young people under conditions of late modernity. The *Journal of Youth Studies* has showcased much of this debate. We see it, for example, in the argument between J. J. Arnett (2006) and John Bynner (2005) about the relative importance of social structure in determining the prevalence, and theoretical novelty, of 'emerging adulthood' as a supposed new life phase. It lies at the heart of the 'post-subcultural' rejection of earlier subculture theory and in the recent to and fro between exponents of the value of each (Bennett 1999, Bennett and Kahn-Harris 2004, Blackman 2005, Hesmondhalgh 2005, Shildrick and MacDonald 2006). Arguments about the extent and consequences of 'individualization' always refer to the perceived role of social class in shaping biographies ('choice' versus 'normal') with influential authors reminding us of the limits placed by social structure, particularly class, on individual choice in their theorizations of 'bounded agency' (Evans 2002) or 'structured individualisation' (Roberts 1995). Beck's theories of 'risk society' and of individualization have had enormous influence in youth studies. Woodman (2009) is perhaps right, however, in his recent defence of Beck that their influence has been seen in good part as a set of ideas to argue against. Rather than the orthodox position in youth studies being the downplaying of social structural divisions, such as social class, and the elevation of individual choice and agency in understanding young people's lives, the opposite is true, argues Woodman.

So, despite the recognition of rapid and widespread processes of globalization, which some argue have diminished the significance of class and place in shaping social life, class still plays a significant role in many attempts to theorize youth. The facts of class and place are hard to ignore when we are faced with statistics that show, for the UK for instance, inequality widening and social mobility stalling (DWP 2009). Class inequality persists in virtually all walks of life (Hills *et al.* 2009). This is all despite British Prime Ministers of different political hues proclaiming, from time to time, the fact of a 'classless society' and the hardening of the attitudes of the British public to those at the bottom. Explanations citing social injustice have declined, and those blaming individual failings have risen over the past 25 years. As Castell and Thompson (2007, p. 7) put it, there is 'still a mountain to climb even just to get people to "base camp" in terms of the causes and consequences of poverty in the UK'. Attempts by the UK New Labour government to eliminate child poverty have faltered, and research highlights the high proportions of children still growing up in conditions of severe poverty and deprivation (DWP 2009). Outcomes for these young, working-class people are almost always worse than for their economically advantaged counterparts (see Shildrick 2008 for a review of some of this recent social policy discussion). The relative political invisibility of New Labour's child poverty targets – and public complacency about their failure to meet them – is further testament to the political lack of interest in or denial of the class problem in Britain.

Youth cultural identities: class, place and space

Theoretical and critical understanding of the politics of place reveals opposing positions. Fredric Jameson (1991, p. 16) sees the spatial logic of capitalism as an organizing tool that shapes and determines the social relations of oppression, while hooks (1991, p. 145) sees the radical potential of new spaces for resistance to struggle for a place to be. In this collection of work on young people, class and place, we can see how young people's experiences are lived at a biographical, cultural and structural level, focusing on cultural practices, new class formations, ethnic and gender relations, and contemporary class struggles. The various contributions address the ways in which young people use different social spaces and subcultural identities to reveal complex social negotiation as they encounter diverse social action within the community. Bell hooks' use of Adrienne Rich's (1984) concept of the 'politics of location' has resonance with youth because young people tend to be positioned as marginal and second-class citizens (Furlong and Cartmel 2007). hooks' focus on social pressures from the border is brought to life in these papers where different young people experience the contradictions of desire, ambition, repression and resistance.

Recent sociological analyses of class outside youth studies have been invigorated by research on the subtle ways in which class is reproduced in contemporary society. The politics of globalization and the postmodern questioning of place have brought opportunities and instabilities in the creation of young people's social class identities. Through the different examples we can see that particular places have meaning and bring a sense of belonging, and a form of space is created through acts of naming and activity via memory. We see young people engaged in forms of reflexivity, where place to adults can appear dangerous and dirty, but to young people their engagement in public space is part of their cultural habitus (Bourdieu 1993).

The paper by Sumi Hollingworth and colleagues is an excellent example of the interest of the 'new working-class studies' in the discursive, psychic and moral landscapes of class (e.g. Sayer 2005, Skeggs 2005); of how social class divisions are felt, seen, used and talked about (if infrequently named directly) by young people in the contexts of contemporary youth cultures and secondary schooling. A critical division emerges, this and other recent studies suggest (McCulloch *et al.* 2006), between most young people and their cultural forms and 'them', the 'chavs'. We interpret the rapid, recent rise in the UK of negative depictions of 'chavs' and 'charvers' (Hayward and Yar 2006) as modern-day echoes of age-old representations of the disorderly and undeserving working class. Popular, everyday talk about 'chavs' can be 'deeply offensive', according to Tom Hampson of the Fabian Society (2007). Calling for class discrimination to be taken more seriously and use of the 'chav' term to be 'banned', he calls this language 'sneering, patronising and dangerous' and aimed at groups who have no political voice. As Tyler (2008, p. 32) concludes in her discussion of the use of the term in respect of young single mothers, 'the cumulative effect of disgust at chavs is the screening of the disenfranchised white poor from view; they are rendered invisible, inaudible or, like Vicky Pollard, laughably incomprehensible'.[2]

What makes the 'chav' or 'charver' discourse so powerful, under the guise of either harmless light entertainment or unreflective, uncritical social science, is its role in pinning the mass of young, poor, white, working-class people to the social pathologies of, *inter alia*, welfare dependency, moral degeneracy, academic failure, fecklessness, and excessive and tasteless consumption as if these were (a) accurate depictions of their life situations, (b) the common problems of all, and (c) rooted in individual failings (Shildrick *et al.* 2007). While offensive, prejudicial language rooted in other social divisions and disadvantage (such as by ethnicity, sexuality, disability, gender) has waned in popular discourse and all but disappeared from academic writing, class prejudice – in the form of 'chav talk' – proliferates in the UK.

These objections are not just rooted in po-faced, 'political correctness'. As Howard Becker (1963) taught us, labels carry meanings and meanings have consequences. This is perhaps most clearly demonstrated in the investigation here by Robert Ralphs and colleagues of the consequences for 'non-gang-affiliated' young people of growing up in places affected by youth gangs. This ethnographic work provides a robust counter to sensationalized and exaggerated depictions of the infestation of British cities by youth gangs. Critically, it reveals the pressures and exclusionary effects of gang labelling on young lives already constrained by the disadvantages of class, place and 'race'. The pincer movement of (mis)labelling and harassment by police and by gang members (and the legal and illegal threats that lent this labelling power) severely curtailed the room for manoeuvre of non-'gang youth' (literally and metaphorically). Being wrongly excluded from school, with serious ramifications for future educational and employment transitions and opportunities, is one example the authors give of the social exclusionary effects of gang labelling on young people. The ultimate form of social exclusion described, however, is of young people being shot dead because of presumed gang affiliations.

Like Ralphs *et al.*, Cara Robinson is also interested in young people's leisure, their use of space and its meanings. More specifically, she has researched close up how a small group of young people in south-east England use public space in their leisure time. An important aspect of this paper, we think, is the sense of normality, the fun and the leisureliness of young people's collective occupation of public space – and the value of this to the experience of being young. Robinson empathetically understands the meaning of space from the point of view of young people, usefully getting behind the usual 'social problem' policy and media accounts that attach to 'youth on the streets'. While 'things happened' (Robinson cites Corrigan's valuable but often overlooked contribution to *Resistance Through Rituals*: Hall and Jefferson 1976), and memories of these events bonded the group in a collective history, readers might get the sense that often not very much happened – at least not in ways dramatic or notable to an interested adult observer. While Robinson, too, is interested in issues of the governance and surveillance of youth and space, the contrast with the sense of danger, entrapment and fear reported by Ralphs and colleagues' research participants is striking. *Where* spaces are, the *places* they are in, and *who* occupies them tell us much about how space is used and its meanings for young people.

Class, youth transitions and place: continuities and change

The nod by Ralphs and colleagues towards the consequences for youth transitions of experiences of place, space, leisure and associated cultural identities is fleshed out in the work by Anthony Gunter and Paul Watt. Their paper is also one that looks ethnographically at young people – in this case, primarily young black men – growing up in a place (east London) that has experienced social change, economic uncertainty and disadvantage. Given UK media obsession with 'the problem' of black young men and youth gangs in London, it is refreshing that gangs are not central to their discussion. Gunter and Watt provide what, unfortunately, still remains a rare example of youth research that integrates 'the two traditions' of UK youth research (Coles 1986, Cohen and Ainley 2000), asking questions about youth leisure, style, and subcultural identity, and questions about youth transitions. Neither, they argue, can be properly answered without reference to the other – nor without reference to the structure of opportunities available in places experiencing global-local socio-economic change (see Nayak 2004, 2006, for another good, recent example). Thus, Gunter and Watt describe three main subcultural formations: 'grafting' (with strong cultural continuities with the 'real', masculine, classed work preferred by Willis's famous working-class 'lads', 1977), 'going to college' (followed by young men and women, and partly influenced by avoidance of 'grafting' culture), and 'going on road' (rejection of the racism and limitations of the labour market, and the pursuit of petty crime and 'badness'). Notably, and unusually, they emphasize how these subcultural styles form in relation to labour market opportunities and transitions and not just in articulation with leisure, music and style.

Charlie Walker's paper sits firmly within the tradition of youth transitions studies. While one of only two papers here that reports research from beyond the UK, it at least helped to some degree in comparative analysis of youth transitions. Walker demonstrates how under processes of economic change the labour market fails to deliver the prospect of successful transitions for many working-class young people. His concerns will be familiar to those interested in processes of youth transition and class dislocation in the West. He conjures with the restructuring and individualization of youth employment and training transitions in radically altered economic circumstances (in post-communist Russia). Despite the geographic and social distance between the place he researched and those of the majority of papers in the collection, we were struck by the continuities and similarities between them in respect of the experiences, motivations and sentiments expressed by young people. In struggling through their changed economic landscape, interviewees sought to make sense of their situations, often in highly individualized ways. As in Gunter and Watt's study – and in studies from Teesside (MacDonald and Marsh 2004) – regrets about lack of effort and achievement at school were common, with individual lack of progress in the labour market frequently theorized in terms of personal 'failure' at school (rather than in terms of the contingencies of class-based and closed-down opportunity structures). This is a clear example of the 'epistemological fallacy' that Furlong and Cartmel (2007) say besets young people under conditions of risk society and individualization.

Continuity and change is the central theme of the paper by Tom Hall and colleagues. There is a tendency in sociology – perhaps particularly in youth studies – to seek out evidence of the new and the different. Less likely to grab the headlines, but perhaps equally interesting, is evidence of the old and the same; of continuity rather than change. Indeed, it is more interesting if circumstances would predict change and discontinuity. As in other papers, Hall and colleagues have undertaken detailed, qualitative research with young people that is strongly attentive to the conditions of the place in which those young people live (in Ebbw Vale, in South Wales – a place of recent dramatic economic upheaval). Unlike the other authors, these authors chose not to report empirical findings in any detail but instead want to reflect on how we think about the transitions of young people in their places. Even in a locality marked by the severe economic shock that came with the closure of the local steelworks (and what this symbolized about the dismantling of traditional working-class transitions to employment and wider forms of community), Hall and colleagues insist on balancing our analytical concern with change, breaks and disruption, with a sense of stability, of lives led day to day, of the phenomenological experience of continuity.

In putting together this volume about class and place, we did not wish to argue that social class divisions might trump other dimensions of social inequality. We suspect it would be difficult to get unanimity between the editors, never mind the authors, on this question, and space, of course, has disallowed authors charged with the task of writing about place and class to say much about how these intersect with, say, issues of gender or ethnicity. We do get glimpses, though. Gunter and Watt focus primarily on the experiences of black young men and note how processes of racist exclusion in part shape the transitions they describe. Although they do not make great play of the fact, Ralphs and colleagues' research questions some common misconceptions about ethnicity and gang membership. Yvette Taylor and Michelle Addison's paper, of all here, gives most consideration to the intertwining of gender and class in its exposition of the meanings of places for women of different ages and classes in north-east England. At first glance, their inclusion of older women in a journal of *youth* studies seems odd. Yet we think that their methodological inclusion of different generations of women from the same localities provides the rare possibility of analysis of continuity and change in women's lives over decades. They research in a region that has undergone profound economic change and in locales within that region that have 'enjoyed' quite different levels and experience of recovery and regeneration. How young women, of different classes, are situated within, relate to, and make sense of this changing, classed landscape of uneven possibilities is the focus of their paper.

Finally, a word about methodological approaches to understanding class, place and youth: all bar one of these papers employ qualitative methods of different varieties to get close to the meanings of class and place as they are lived by young people. The lens is highly focused. As advocates and practitioners of qualitative research with young people, we are naturally heartened to see the vitality of research of this sort, and the insights they bring. Gone are the days when critics could complain about the hegemony of 'dry', quantitative, policy-dominated mappings of youth transitions in youth studies (Miles 2000). Nonetheless, we are disappointed that there were few submissions to consider for publication that used alternative, particularly quantitative methodologies, but pleased to be able to include at least one fine example that reports very important findings. Ken Roberts and Gary Pollock examine emerging new class divisions in the new market economies of the south Caucasus through large-scale surveying of the longitudinal, biographical experiences of the first post-communist cohorts of young adults in these countries. This wider lens allows the authors to ask and answer different sorts of questions from those of the other papers: about longer and broader processes of class formation as revealed by youth transitions in states themselves undergoing transition. Their paper, as all do, point up paths of continuity and change with the past and, in this case, lines of connection in processes of the shaping of class at global level, between East and

West. It also returns us to our starting point; the privileged vantage point of youth studies in seeing patterns of social change and reproduction of significance beyond the realms of youth studies

Notes

1. Marx and Engels (1848: 80–83), *The Communist Manifesto.*
2. 'Vicky Pollard' is presented as a comical character in the BBC television comedy series, *Little Britain.*

References

Arnett, J., 2006. Emerging adulthood in Britain: a response to Bynner. *Journal of youth studies*, 9 (1), 111–123.
Becker, H.S., 1963. *Outsiders.* New York: Free Press.
Bennett, A., 1999. Sub-cultures or neo-tribes? Rethinking the relationship between youth style and musical taste. *Sociology*, 33 (3), 599–617.
Bennett, A., 2005. In defence of neo-tribes: a response to Blackman and Hesmondhalgh. *Journal of youth studies*, 8 (1), 255–259.
Bennett, A. and Kahn-Harris, K., eds. 2004. *After subculture.* London: Palgrave.
Blackman, S., 2005. Youth subcultural theory: a critical engagement with the concept, its origins and politics, from the Chicago School to post modernism. *Journal of youth studies*, 8 (1), 1–20.
Bourdieu, P., 1993. *The field of cultural production.* Cambridge: Polity Press.
Bynner, J., 2005. Rethinking the youth phase: the case for emerging adulthood? *Journal of youth studies*, 8 (4), 367–384.
Byrne, D., 2005. *Social exclusion.* Maidenhead: Open University Press.
Castell, S. and Thompson, J., 2007. *Understanding attitudes to poverty in the UK.* York: Joseph Rowntree Foundation.
Castells, M., 1989. *The informational city.* Oxford: Basil Blackwell.
Cohen, P. and Ainley, P., 2000. In the country of the blind? Youth studies and cultural studies in Britain. *Journal of youth studies*, 3 (1), 79–95.
Coles, B., 1986. 'Gonna tear your playhouse down': towards reconstructing a sociology of youth. *Social science teacher*, 15 (3), 178–180.
Corrigan, P., 1976. Doing nothing. *In*: S. Hall and T. Jefferson, eds. *Resistance through rituals.* London: Hutchinson, 103–105.
DWP, 2009. *The living standards of families with children reporting low incomes.* Department of Work and Pensions (DWP), research report no. 577. London: DWP.
Evans, K., 2002. Taking control of their lives? Agency in young adult transitions in England and the new Germany. *Journal of youth studies*, 5 (3), 245–270.
Furlong, A. and Cartmel, F., 2007. *Young people and social change.* Milton Keynes: Open University Press.
Hampson, T., 2007. *Stop using chav.* London: Fabian Society.
Harvey, D., 2005. *The new imperialism.* New York: Oxford University Press.
Hayward, K. and Yar, M., 2006. The "chav" phenomenon: consumption, media and the construction of a new underclass. Crime, media. *culture*, 2 (1), 9–28.
Hesmondhalgh, D., 2005. Subcultures, scenes or tribes? None of the above. *Journal of youth studies*, 8 (1), 21–40.
Hills, J., Sefton, T., and Stewart, K., 2009. *Towards a more equal society.* Bristol: Policy Press.
Hooks, B., 1991. *Yearning: race, gender and cultural politics.* London: Turnaround.
Jameson, F., 1991. *Postmodernism: the cultural logic of late capitalism.* London: Verso.
Jeffs, T. and Smith, M., 1998. The problem of "youth" for youth work. *Youth and policy*, 62, 45–66.
MacDonald, R. and Marsh, J., 2004. Missing school. *Youth and society*, 36 (2), 143–162.
MacDonald, R. and Shildrick, T., 2009. Youth sub-culture, youth transitions and youth studies: some reflections on 'the state of play'. ESRC Rethinking Youth Cultures in the Age of Global Media research seminar series, Institute of Education, London.

Marx, K., 1887/1954. *Capital*, vol. 1. London: Lawrence and Wishart.
Marx, K. and Engels, F., 1848/2009. *The Communist Manifesto.* Harmondsworth: Penguin.
McCulloch, K., Stewart, A., and Lovegreen, N., 2006. 'We just hang out together': youth cultures and social class. *Journal of youth studies*, 9 (5), 539–556.
Miles, S., 2000. *Youth lifestyles in a changing world.* Buckingham: Open University Press.
Nayak, A., 2004. *Race, place and globalization.* Oxford: Berg.
Nayak, A., 2006. Displaced masculinities: chavs, youth and class in the post-industrial city. *Sociology*, 40 (5), 813–831.
Rich, A., 1984/86. Notes towards a politics of location. *In*: *Blood, bread and poetry: selected prose 1979–1985.* New York: W.W. Norton, 210–231.
Roberts, K., 1995. *Youth and employment in modern Britain.* Oxford: Oxford University Press.
Sayer, A., 2005. *The moral significance of class.* Cambridge: Cambridge University Press.
Shildrick, T., 2008. Hiding out in the open: young people and social class in UK youth studies. *Youth and Policy*, 100, 205–213.
Shildrick, T. and MacDonald, R., 2006. In defence of subculture: young people, leisure and social divisions. *Journal of youth studies*, 9 (2), 125–140.
Shildrick, T., MacDonald, R. and Webster, C., 2006. Class, consumption and prejudice: contemporary representations of "the social scum". ESRC Consumption and Identities research seminar series, University of Teesside.
Skeggs, B., 2005. *Class, self and culture.* London: Routledge.
Skeggs, B, Thumim, N., and Wood, H., 2008. Oh goodness, I'm watching reality TV: how methods makes class in audience research. *European journal of cultural studies*, 11 (5), 1–21.
Tyler, I., 2008. Chav mum, chav scum': class disgust in contemporary Britain. *Feminist media studies*, 8 (1), 17–34.
Willis, P., 1977. *Learning to labour.* Farnborough: Saxon House.
Woodman, D., 2009. The mysterious case of the pervasive choice biography: Ulrich Beck, structure/agency, and the middling state of theory in the sociology of youth. *Journal of youth studies*, 12 (3), 243–256.

Constructions of the working-class 'Other' among urban, white, middle-class youth: 'chavs', subculture and the valuing of education

Sumi Hollingworth and Katya Williams

Institute for Policy Studies in Education, London Metropolitan University, London, UK

In the context of a 'death' of class in popular and policy discourse, this paper argues that social class is still a major force at work in young people's lives, particularly in the context of schooling. We argue that young people's subcultural groups are classed, in the way in which they are constructed in discourse. Drawing on a data set of 68 interviews with white, middle-class young people in three different cities in England, we argue that class can be seen and felt in young people's constructions of the 'chav', where white, working-class young people's ways of being and doing in the context of schooling, stand in stark contrast to the normative middle-class subject, and become pathologized.

Introduction

This paper, drawing on 'cultural' class analyses in the sociology of education, aims to contribute to a growing body of work in youth studies seeking to place class back on the agenda (see, for example, McCulloch *et al.* 2006, Shildrick and MacDonald 2006). Education is one area where researchers have maintained a small but consistent spotlight on the 'injuries' of class (Sennett and Cobb 1972), and in Britain socio-economic background is still the biggest predictor of educational success or failure (Office for National Statistics 2005). Within youth studies there has been a recent move to foreground the importance of social class in the study of youth (McCulloch *et al.* 2006, Nayak 2006, Shildrick and MacDonald 2006), stressing that young people's subcultural styles and identities are still closely bound up with social class. 'Post-subcultural' studies have tended to take an approach that emphasizes individualism and consumer lifestyle youth affiliations (see Redhead 1990, Thornton 1995, Miles 2000), stressing the '*loosening* of social structures such as social class' (McCulloch *et al.* 2006, p. 542). However, the social geographer Nayak (2003, p. 320) has argued that young people's cultural identities continue to be 'closely intertwined with family histories, gender, place, class, region and locality'. Hence, Shildrick and MacDonald (2006) have argued for a return to a classed analysis of youth subcultural groupings. They argue that 'youth culture' studies could learn something from 'youth transitions' research (for example, Furlong and Cartmel 1997, Ball *et al.* 2000, MacDonald *et al.* 2005), which tends to be more aware of the structural inequalities in young people's lives. Not all young people are able to create cultural identities in the same way (Shildrick and MacDonald 2006, p. 131), and, as feminist education research has demonstrated, different cultural identities (which are classed, raced and gendered) carry unequal value or worth (Skeggs 2004, Archer *et al.* 2007).

This renewed focus on class in academic study operates as a response to a general decline in the use of the term in political and popular speak in Britain, where there is a closing down of public welfare discourses, increasingly replaced with a language of social exclusion (Whitty 2001, McDowell 2006, Reay 2006), in which individuals are increasingly seen as responsible for their own success, and structural constraints such as class, gender and race are downplayed. Critics argue that contemporary policy is based on a particular model of the (individualized) self as enterprising, reflexive, autonomous and self-regulating, and the failure to enact this 'normative selfhood' is explained as (social exclusion and) the outcome of individual pathology (Lawler 2005, Allen 2008).

A cultural approach to class

In our analysis we take the view that 'economic conditions constitute just one aspect of class rather than providing us with a comprehensive picture' (Archer and Francis 2006, p. 140). We work with a broader notion of social class that encompasses how class may be grounded within and produced through people's identities and cultural practices, rather than just their occupational backgrounds. We take the position that classed identities are not always fixed, but can be defined through practices and process (Skeggs 2004, p. 151). Skeggs (2005, p. 965) argues that in the contemporary discourse, 'class is rarely named directly but connoted through "moral euphemism" whereby processes of interpretation do the work of association.' Following Skeggs (2004), we highlight the importance of representation – the way in which, particularly, certain working-class groups come to be represented by more dominant groups and the very real effects of this.

In this paper we examine the 'talk' of a sample of middle-class young people in schools in three cities, and the ways in which classed boundaries or borders are constructed and maintained. Thorne (1993) uses the term 'border work' to describe the maintenance of gender boundaries among schoolchildren, and we find it useful to explore the ways in which discourses of subculture (and particularly the 'chav') are used by our middle-class sample to create classed boundaries between 'us and them' (Southerton 2002). Drawing on the work of Frederik Barth, Thorne argues, 'one can gain insight into the maintenance of ethnic (and gender) [and we would argue, class] groups by examining the boundary that defines them rather than by looking at what Barth calls "the cultural stuff that it encloses".' (Thorne 1993, p. 65, citing Barth 1969, p. 15). Following on from this assertion, in this paper we use Andrew Sayer's (2005) analysis of the way in which classed boundaries are constructed along three main lines: aesthetic (regarding matters such as décor, clothing and appearance), performative (regarding behaviour and performance), and moral (regarding values), though of course these categories overlap.

We argue that where class is concerned, this border work is heavily grounded in moral judgements, which involves a process of 'othering', in which the middle classes assert their moral worth by ascribing negative characteristics to the working-class 'Other' (see Skeggs 2005, p. 977). As Lawler suggests, one way in which class inequality is reproduced is through processes of 'making working class subjectivities pathological, so that class relations are not just economic relations but also relations of superiority/inferiority, normality/abnormality, judgment/shame' (Lawler, 1999, p. 4, cited in Tyler and Bennett forthcoming, p. 3). Specifically, we seek to contribute to such empirical analyses of how 'chav' operates within wider circuits of class making.

After providing some brief details of the empirical research on which this paper is based, we turn to a general discussion of the young people's talk about youth subcultural groupings in their schools, exploring regional differences in our data, but maintaining a focus on the classed and raced dynamics of these. We then move on to focus more substantively on 'talk' about chavs and charvers, deconstructing how they are discussed in three main ways, by their appearance (aesthetic), their behaviour (performative), and their values (moral), and we examine the ways in which this is a form of 'border work' which sets them up as a pathologized group. We finish by discussing the messiness of the class boundaries in the young people's talk, arguing that despite young people's assertions that chavs do not map simply onto working-class groups, this is still an identity they wish to avoid.

The study

This paper is drawing on findings from an ESRC study[1] in which we interviewed white, urban, middle-class families who chose to send their children to the local inner-city comprehensive school.[2] Urban state schools in Britain have often had a bad reputation (Ward 1990 [1978]), and it is common for the middle classes living in cities to send their children to private or academically selective state schools or 'play the system' to get their children into the 'better' comprehensive schools, such as moving house to be in the catchment area (Ball 2003, Butler and Robson 2003). This then leaves non-selective state schools in inner-city areas with predominantly working-class populations (Reay 2004).[3] It is argued that one reason for clamouring for the 'better' schools is related to fears about whom their children will be mixing with (Byrne 2006). As we will show, these fears were also present in the families in our study, who made a positive choice of their local comprehensive school. The study focused on their motivations and commitments and the way in which choice of the local school might be related to particular identities or identifications. We asked the parents and their children about their experiences of the school, their grades, and their aspirations. We also specifically talked to parents and their children about the extent to which they mixed with young people from other social and ethnic backgrounds and how they felt about this.

This research involved interviews with 124 families (180 individual interviews with mothers or fathers and 68 individual interviews with children). The research focused on three cities in England: London, a north-east city that we have called 'Norton', and a south-west city that we have called 'Riverton'.[4] We draw predominantly on the data set of 68 interviews with the young people in the families (supplemented by some extracts from their parents' interviews where illustrative). The young people we spoke to were aged between 12 and 25 (so some were talking about their previous experiences of attending an inner-city comprehensive, but the majority were still attending their school).[5]

Youth subcultural groups and class

Tyler (2006) and Skeggs (2004) have previously argued that in the media, class is often referred to in euphemistic terms (and see Bromley 2000). This 'classless' rhetoric was quite apparent in our sample across the three cities. For the young people in our research, boundaries were often drawn more implicitly, along the lines of music tastes and fashion tastes; however, in line with recent assertions in youth studies (McCulloch *et al.* 2006, Nayak 2006, Shildrick and MacDonald 2006), we argue that social class divisions are evident in this. Nayak (2006, p. 828) asserts:

> [. . .]while social class may rarely be discussed directly by young people it continues to be threaded through the daily fabric of their lives: it is stitched into codes of respect, accent, dress, music, bodily adornment and comportment. In short, the affective politics of class is a felt practice, tacitly understood and deeply internalized.

Nayak implies that while social class is not really a concept that young people use, it is visible in their subcultural groupings. A quotation from one of the young women in our research, Rhiannon Foster (aged 16, from Redwood School in Riverton), gives weight to this notion that subcultural divisions are so tacit yet deeply internalized:

> It's really hard to describe because when you're in it, you understand it perfectly, but talking to people about it, it's really hard to put it into words because everybody knows it.

McCulloch and colleagues' (2006) empirical research on youth subcultures in Edinburgh and Newcastle found that the different groups ('goths', 'skaters' and 'charvers/Neds') mapped, to a large extent, on to classed divisions, though the young people did not refer to them as such. They found in terms of parental occupation, the charvers clustered around lower social classes, with none at all in the professional and managerial categories, while goths and skaters showed a wider range of backgrounds, but were more likely to belong to higher social classes. Similarly the goths and skaters were all in full-time education or employment, while the charvers were predominantly unemployed (McCulloch *et al.* 2006, p. 552).

In our research the young people similarly told us about the different subcultural groupings in the school, such as 'hippies' or 'poshies' (Norton), 'goths' and 'emos' (Norton and Riverton), 'skaters' or 'jitters' (Norton and Riverton), 'rockers' and 'gangsters' (London), and 'townies' or 'chavs' or 'charvers' (predominantly Norton and Riverton). In line with McCulloch *et al.*'s (2006) work, these groups often did not label themselves as such and the names are those given by others. The white middle classes in our sample unanimously told us they tended to be labelled by others as hippies or poshies, or jitters or rockers, but never chavs, townies or gangsters.

The reason for these labels, they told us, was often due to their 'posh' accent, their long hair (hippies or rockers), and their choice of alternative or independent rock music (jitters, rockers) and associated clothing. There are obvious class connotations to these groupings in school, with the term 'poshies' denoting middle or upper classness, and 'hippies' having their roots in middle-class radicalism (Parkin 1968). William Smart, aged 15, at Meadowood School in Riverton, also referred to the 'emos' in classed terms, claiming they are 'whingey . . . white urban middle class kids'. As McCulloch *et al.* (2006) found, our young people talked about how chavs were from poorer backgrounds and areas. Chavs were seen to come from 'deprived areas' of the city (Toby Webb, aged 12, The Park School, Norton) or were 'people on benefits' (Jill Cole, aged 18, Wordsworth School, Norton), and some even named specific areas of the city known for socio-economic deprivation. A few, when asked to describe 'chav', named it specifically as 'working class'.

Subcultural groups and ethnicity

There was little mention of chavs in London, whereas in Norton and Riverton popular pathologizing discourses of chavs or charvers were common. In London, depictions of the working classes were complicated by ethnicity, which seemed to be the overriding factor in terms of different subcultural groups. To give some context: while the vast majority of schools in all the cities had higher than average proportions of children receiving free school meals (an indication of poverty levels), in every London school we cite in this paper, white British pupils make up the minority, black and minority ethnic pupils making up 60–90 per cent of the school. However, in nearly all of the schools in Norton and Riverton, white children made up the majority. Davina Cunningham, aged 18, at Saint Thomas' School in London, for example, explained about her school:

> There was just a culture there [. . .] like there were people from loads of different ethnic groups. You would have the Latin American groups and they would cause a bit of trouble and then you would have the Caribbean groups and they would cause a bit of trouble, each would have like their own sections of the playground as well.

A few of the young people in London talked about 'gangs' in their school, and gang membership seemed to revolve around both ethnicity, and local area affiliation. Noah Mallone, aged 15, at Springdale School in London, told us, 'There is like a big black gang, loads of Bengali gangs', and in his school, Hetherington in London, Zach Watson, aged 14, talked about how rivalry was often 'Turks versus blacks'. This was also connected to which area of the city you lived in.

As we have discussed elsewhere (Reay *et al.* 2007), we argue that in London, the presence of larger numbers of minority ethnic young people in the schools almost acts as a 'buffer zone' between the white middle classes and their classed Other, the white working classes. We could argue the difference results from different discursive framings within dominant discourses of neoliberal multiculturalism in London (see Haylett 2001, p. 365), where multicultural friendships, or mix, is celebrated as a key aspect of a particularly kind of London middle-class lifestyle (see, for example, May 1996, Haylett 2001, Byrne 2006), while in all three cities there was little valuing of white, working-class culture or cross-class friendship (see Reay *et al.* 2007).

The white middle classes as 'outsiders'

Several parents described how their children's school was divided by the different subcultural groups. Gemma Foster, aged 13, explained how in her school (Redwood) in Riverton, 'generally you stick to your own groups'. One mother (Angela Gordon, Norton) told us, 'There's a sort of division in school between the charvs and [my son and daughter] get called the 'hippies' or the 'poshies'.' In a process of boundary making (Southerton 2002) or 'border work' (Thorne 1993), young people in Norton and Riverton were keen to define themselves in opposition to the charvers. One mother (Anne Downie, in Norton) explained about her daughter, 'She's um part of an interesting little [laughs] friendship group, who define themselves as non-charvers.' In this sense, the charvers are a constitutive 'Other', against which the middle class constitutes the self as respectable (Skeggs 2004; also see Crozier *et al.* 2008). This is something we will explore further, later in the paper. Similarly, Noah Mallone, aged 15, at Springdale school in London, was keen to assert that he and his friends were not chavs or gangsters, but nor were they geeks:

> Our group is kind of like the outsiders but not the geeks in a way. We are kind of like ... basically most of our school is just chavs and just people who think they are gangsters and they are not.

He explained that these 'gangs' were into gangster rap and grime music, whereas his group were 'just kind of mostly rockers'. In several schools in both Norton and Riverton, young people reported that chavs made up the majority. Todd Western, aged 18, Marley School, London, which had 90 per cent Asian pupils, told us, 'I always felt a bit out of place there' because he was the only one who listened to heavy metal music. Similarly, Frankie Cadogan, aged 18, Eastleigh Common School, London, who had moved from school to a college in the other side of London, admitted that at school 'everyone was just sort of different' from him and were into 'different stuff' such as listening to rap and R&B, whereas he liked to listen to rock and 'old music' like Pink Floyd.

When asked more explicitly about the extent to which these lifestyle differences were classed and raced, Todd admitted that 'most of my people who are into what I'm into are white', and 'at the moment my friends are mainly white.' Frankie claimed that young people in his school were different from him because it was a predominantly working-class school, and they were the kinds of people who had never left the local area, whereas he had American parentage and was well travelled. Noah, however, rejected the suggestion that subcultural groups in his school fell along class and race lines, claiming the divisions were more to do with behaviour and engagement with education, a discussion we will return to later.

Like Noah, many of the young people we spoke to saw themselves as outside the usual groups in the school. Toby Webb's (aged 12, The Park School, Norton) assertion was common one:

> I don't like carrying that sort of name, I think it's silly being classified into a group of people because I just like being myself.

While the working classes in the school were fixed by place by their local regional accent and their lack of mobility, and were labelled chavs, gangsters and townies, the middle classes were free-floating, asserting independence from such labels.

Chavs and charvers

We argue that in Norton and Riverton there are much smaller proportions of ethnic minorities to provide a 'protective barrier' (compared to London). Thus we would argue that it is the white working classes who were more denigrated, labelled as chavs or charvers, and were seen to constitute more of the threat to the white middle classes (see Reay *et al.* 2007). Sayer (2005a) also claims that this border work is 'particularly strong in groups that are anxious about their position' in relation to those who are above and those who are below (see also Raisborough and Adams 2008).

Proliferation and repetition of class markers might point towards a perceived fragility of the presence and position of the white middle class in Norton: 'if they were secure, differences would not need to be continually drawn, values established, legitimated and institutionalized' (Skeggs 2004, p. 117). We now turn to discuss the border work involved in the othering of chavs and charvers.

It is important to draw attention to the wider context. As we have highlighted in the beginning of this paper, the term 'chav' (with regional variation 'charv' or 'charver') has become popularized across the country (Hayward and Yar 2006, Tyler 2006). The people we interviewed do not exist in a vacuum, they are situated and influenced by surrounding discourses. Wetherell and Potter refer to this as 'interpretative repertoires': broadly discernible clusters of terms, descriptions and figures of speech often assembled around metaphors or vivid images (1992, p. 90). As Sayer highlights, in making judgements actors draw upon 'available ways of thinking about such matters' (2005b, p. 142), including not only moral norms but discourses such as those of racism, sexism and class, and 'chav' seemed to be the main available discourse to discuss social difference in Norton and Riverton.

As Holt and Griffin argue, 'Othering enables the middle classes to focus on aspects of their identities which they wish to hold up as defining their groups' characteristics (e.g. middle class taste, intelligence, refinement), while denying these characteristic to the working class Other' (2005, p. 248). As Bourdieu puts it, 'taste classifies and it classifies the classifier' (Bourdieu 1984, p. 56). We could see how the charvers were defined by a distinct set of characteristics that were denigrated by parents and children alike. Andrew Sayer's (2005b) three categories become particularly relevant here. These denigrated characteristics were aesthetic, performative and moral. Chavs were most commonly defined by their brash and excessive dress and appearance (aesthetic); their careless, unruly and often violent behaviour (performative); and, in the context of schooling, their lack of respect for and disengagement with education (moral), as we will now explain. In many cases this border work in young people's discourses was not clear-cut and did not necessarily map exactly onto class or ethnic groups; but we argue, nevertheless, that these discourses serve to essentialize the white working classes and is classed in the consequences.

Aesthetic boundaries: 'chavs' and their appearance

In line with popular conceptions (Hayward and Yar 2006), many of the young people interviewed described charvers by the clothes they wear. This usually centred on lots of jewellery, tracksuits, and certain designer brands, such as Burberry, Rockport, Kappa, Berghaus, Lacoste. Class was read into these fashion styles by some: as one mother described in her child's school, 'You could tell from external factors like the style of dress [. . .] it clearly wasn't middle class.'

In line with Skeggs' analysis of representations of the working classes, the language used was a language of excess, or what Tyler and Bennett (forthcoming) refer to as 'excessive corporeality'. The young people asserted, 'They wear like *massive* rings all over their hands'; 'they wear usually like a *big* coat like as a statement like with a *big* collar, usually a Berghaus, and they wear peak caps and that, and they just, they wear like Rockports, and they all wear *big* shoes and stuff' (James Gordon, age 12, The Park School, Norton). Note the emphasis on 'big':

massive rings, big shoes and big collars. Skeggs (2004) describes Tasker's (1998) research in Hollywood, where she argues that obvious excessive attention to appearance denotes low moral value. There are also clear judgements of taste going on here, as Jay Dunn, aged 12, also at The Park, in Norton, claimed, 'It's a bit tacky as well', and he describes how these young people wear 'scary jewellery and everything'. Jay's description of 'tacky' and Anne Downie's (Norton) comment that they wear 'fake' designer clothing implies an inferior taste, and scary jewellery again emphasizes excess; such excessive jewellery is frightening.

Performative boundaries: 'chavs' and their behaviour

While dress was often the initial point of reference used by these white, middle-class young people, this was often infused with comments about behaviour. Difference was understood or represented as 'spectacle'. This was about being loud and brash, but also being tough and getting into fights, and other, often violent, criminal behaviour. Skeggs (2004) claims that some of the popular ways of representing the working class are as escapist, as dangerous, and as unruly and without shame, and such depictions were reflected in how the charvers were discussed by our participants. This is in direct opposition to depictions of the neo-liberal, rational, bourgeois self as enterprising, reflexive, autonomous and self-regulating (Allen 2008).

Maya Gott, aged 13, at the Edgecliffe School, in Norton, asserts, 'They just, they're like loud and they think they're great and they're just generally annoying'; Natasha Hann, aged 17, at The Park School in Norton, similarly claimed, 'They're very sort of loud and overconfident.' However, interestingly, she asserts that they are loud, 'but in a very different way than the people that I was talking about in private schools.' So these people are loud but in an illegitimate way. For Bourdieu, taste is defined by those who have the power to make their judgements legitimate (Bourdieu 1984), and Natasha recognizes that private school types can also be overconfident, but with more legitimacy. As Skeggs (2004, p. 104) argues, 'respectable excess' is the domain of the middle classes: contained excess is acceptable within limits if practised by those who are seen to be capable of self-governance and restraint.

The young people appeared frightened by this behaviour, but there was also a moral undertone; they looked down on them because they would never engage in such behaviour themselves. Toby Webb, aged 12, at The Park School in Norton, reveals how he also has grown up to see the charvers as 'pathetic':

> I take the mick out of them behind their back because I think it's just incredibly pathetic that you'd want to start a fight with someone really. [. . .] If they're going to be horrible [. . .] if they can't be bothered with school, um, it's just them that's going to end up being a dustbin man or working at the till at some sort of shop when they're older. So I just think of that and [. . .] just let it go.

Toby's comment has connotations of condescension and superiority – he comforts himself with the knowledge that these 'nasty people' will never go far in life, unlike him. We can see here the way in which the othering of the charvers as defined by their violence, bad behaviour, crass taste in clothing, and lack of interest or ability in education favourably positions the middle classes as well behaved, with the 'right taste' and natural educational ability. In addition, in the way in which Toby constructs the chav, we can see elements of mockery, which Raisborough and Adams argue is a way of 'doing' class distinction work under conditions of anxious proximity, in a way which makes the sentiments non-threatening (Raisborough and Adams 2008). However, infusing Toby's talk are notions of 'responsibilisation' (Rose 1996). The chav's failure to enact 'normative selfhood' is constructed as individual pathology (Allen 2008): if chavs choose this behaviour, they will end up in low-status occupations, and this will be their own doing.

Moral boundaries: 'chavs' not valuing education

Paul Willis' (1977) seminal text on working-class masculinity in schools describes the working-class 'lads' who are not interested in school, are disruptive in class, and enjoy having a 'laff' instead.[6] In Norton and Riverton today, chavs and charvers are defined by their disruptiveness in class and reluctance to learn. In a very similar way to how the 'ear'oles' in Willis' study (the more academically committed, working-class pupils in the school) were irritated by the 'lads', the white middle classes in our study were critical of the charvers' behaviour. Rosie Steadman, aged 15, at The Park School in Norton, claimed that in school charvers 'always try and disobey rules and everything', and Jay Dunn, aged 12 in the same school in Norton, claimed that charvers are the ones who are disruptive in class, 'trying to make everyone's life a misery'. Similarly, in Riverton, Rhiannon Foster, aged 16, described how in her school 'Redwood people were [. . .] sometimes more disruptive.' Redwood is where several of the young people claimed chavs or townies come from.

The charvers in school were defined as the ones who 'mess about' and disrupt classes and essentially do not value education. Eleanor Downie, aged 15, at Hillcrest School in Norton, told us:

> [They] often don't come into school if they can't be bothered, and don't really try very hard. [. . .] Um, they're often like naughty in lessons and they just don't do their homework, and always getting into arguments with teachers, and then if they get detentions they don't turn up, so they get one again. They never have their planner or anything with them.

There are a range of moral judgements at work here where the working-class Other is deemed not to be interested in education, not trying, arguing and disrespecting the rules. Eleanor claimed she made a concerted effort to separate herself from these young people. Similarly, Laila Bailey, aged 15, at Rivermead School in Riverton, admitted that she avoided getting in with 'the wrong crowd' that 'mess around in lessons', are 'arrogant' to teachers, and 'don't want to learn'.

We can also see these kinds of moral evaluations (not applying oneself, disrespecting authority, not valuing education) as doing work to set up the chav as in opposition to the middle-class (or 'bourgeois' (Allen 2008)) project of self-making: a moral project in which the self has to show itself to be proper and good, as an object to be worked on (Foucault 1979, Skeggs *et al.* 2007). Skeggs (2007, p. 3) claims that

> one of the main processes by which the 'subject of value' can be distinguished from its constitutive limit is via the amount of labour that is made evident in its making. As a moral imperative people have to show that they are working on their own development, establishing value in their own subjectivity, extending their cultural exchange value.

This, we can argue, underpins middle-class investment in education: they are accruing value (and becoming a 'better' person) through education and credentials, which is an investment for the future. The chavs, on the other hand, are depicted as not investing in the 'self' by sabotaging their education.

Identities related to education were so central to the construction of the charver that there was a sense that real charvers are inherently disinterested and disengaged from education, and if they are successful in education, then they are not 'proper' charvers. Tyler analyses how popular chav celebrities are often the focus of class hatred as they are often constructed as 'the undeserving recipients of wealth': 'the undeserving poor' (Tyler 2008). Here, chavs are constructed as those who are undeserving of educational success. This is expressed well by a conversation with Lucy Gordon, aged 14, at The Park School in Norton, about ability grouping ('setting') in the school. When we asked, 'Are there any charvers in the top sets, then?', she replied that there might be a couple who looked like charvers but because they were 'nice' and in the top set she didn't think they were.

Defining subcultures: struggling with essentialism

As we have noted, subcultural groups did not map clearly onto social class and ethnicity. When asked about whether the different social groupings in school (chav, goth, emo) is about social class, many of the young people (and their parents) denied that this has anything to do with social class, in a move which individualized the phenomenon (Allen 2008). A mother, Jenny Sower, in Norton claimed:

> Whether somebody's a goth or a charv [has] nothing to do with class or background – it's just the sort of people they are really. Um, certainly, my daughter said that some of her old friends from Birchwood Primary were in a group that she wouldn't really mix with now, but that was nothing to do with class – it's, you know, the way they dress, or the sort of music they like [laughs], or something like that.

Martha Redford, aged 16, Gorges School, Riverton, similarly rejected the suggestion that subcultural groups are classed, claiming that it is essentially about personality. Noah Mallone, aged 15, Springdale School, London, also told me that it was simplistic to attribute these differences to social class, but claimed that this division was related to achievement and engagement with school. He claimed that the gangsters and chavs in his school are the people who do not work hard, while his group of friends get on with their schoolwork and are 'not trying to be cool by not working or whatever'. However, this has classed implications, as socio-economic background is a large predictor of educational achievement (Office for National Statistics 2005).

Defining chavs and charvers

The construction of the chav or charver, in particular, was messy and hard to define by these young people. There was a lot of complexity in our data around defining exactly what a charver is. The label was often assigned to young people from working-class areas, but was also highly contingent on disengagement from education. In some cases, chav was described as an identity that you can move in and out of. As we noted, chavs were often described as working class, or coming from 'disadvantaged' homes or 'deprived areas', but young people struggled with the age-old dilemma of structure versus agency in their talk. Jill Cole, aged 18, Wordsworth School, Norton, claimed:

> Um, well, the ones I knew came from Tivton which – Tivton's well known for people being on benefits and just generally not having jobs. Um, I don't think that has anything to do with the way they act though. Um, 'cos my dad was on [benefits], and I didn't act like that. Um, so I don't know, just ...

She claimed that they tend to be people on benefits but is aware that people on benefits are not always charvers. William Greensit, aged 16, Barchester High School, Norton, admitted that 'They're all kind of, kind of generalized – they're all classed as, um, kind of working class and useless and horrible', but he asserted that 'it is true of some people but that's true of some people in a lot of other groups as well.'

In some cases, chav was almost described as an identity that you can buy into. Lots of the young people talked about other children who masquerade as chavs – they are somehow not authentic chavs. Oliver Todd, aged 18, The Shires School, Norton, talked about 'half charvs'; these are people, he explained, who come from nice homes, but socialize with rough people (presumably 'real' charvs). Maya Gott, aged 13, Edgecliffe School, in Norton, struggled over authenticity, claiming that her school is full of 'wannabe charvers' who are merely 'fashion charvers', simply adopting the fashion styles, like Noah Mallone in London, who talked about the 'wannabe' gangsters in his school, people who are not 'real' gangsters. Jill Smith, a mother in Norton, claimed: 'I think, you know, they can all *do* the charver [. . .] and there are almost hierarchies within the charvers – there are posh charvers, there are dangerous charvers, there are, you know, scary charvers [. . .]'. In a similar way to the young men in Nayak's (2006, p. 821) research, who dabble in charver tastes and styles, there is a sense that, in addition to being a label for the white working classes of Norton, chav is also a lifestyle that you can buy into, but at the same time you are not authentic unless you are proper poor, and, of course, it is not a lifestyle they would wish to buy into. The notion that this particular identity position is a *choice* allows for a 'blame the victim' discourse in which, if children choose to be a charv or a gangster, then it is essentially their own fault if they experience the educational consequences of this 'choice' (Allen 2008). It also negates the fact that some people have more power to 'choose' and to reject this identity and hence this label (Archer *et al.* 2007).

Oliver Todd in Norton used the terms 'working class' and 'charv' interchangeably, and when we asked whether charvers were working class, he replied:

> Like not all of them, that's the thing. [. . .] It's just as superficial as any other sort of classification like a hippy or a – it doesn't matter what, like, class you're from, like, anybody can be – I would say, like the majority of people, the majority of charvs probably are like sort of working class, but I wouldn't, I don't really like to say that 'cos it sounds stupid.

Similarly, Emma Greensit, aged 14, Barchester High, Norton, was cautious in defining charvers: 'Um, some of them can actually be very nice, but in general I don't really know them.' She explained:

> Um, I don't like sort of labelling people, kind of going, oh yeah, she's a charver. [. . .] Some people are just, might be called a charver but some are nice and kind, but you get that in every group, you get, you know, hippies who are horrible, whatever – it just happens all the time.

Emma was quick to recognize and assert that there are good and bad people in every social group. Tony Webb, Norton, agreed: 'You can't really generalize about people, because unless they've actually done something to you, you shouldn't really say anything about them.'

Some of the young people in this research rejected such labelling discourses about chavs and charvers. For example, Natasha Hann, aged 17, in Norton, noted that her school experience

> sort of made me realize that, you know, nobody sort of lives up to the stereotypes that you have of them and there's always exceptions and stuff, and you can't just categorize people into groups because like all the people, like even the people that I would sort of see as, you know, complete charvers and stuff, they're not always like that. And you know, I've realized, you know, you can have conversations with people that you just, you just wouldn't think you'd have anything in common with and stuff.

William Smart, aged 15, in Riverton, also told us that he did not like using the term 'chav' because it is 'classist'.

Maintaining a separation

There was a recognition that not all working-class groups are charvers, and that there are 'nice' people and 'nasty' people in all groups. However, this group of white middle-class young people still did not see this lifestyle as something suitable for people like them. It was still necessary to maintain these borders between 'us and them' (Southerton 2002). Many of the young people admitted that they did not mix with charvers or people who came from the 'not nice areas' or people who were disruptive in class. For example, Rhiannon Foster, aged 16, at Redwood School in Riverton, claimed, 'They're not my type of people.' Emma Greensit, aged 14, Barchester High, Norton, claimed not to really know people like that, and others said that they tried to keep away from these kinds of people. James Gordon, age 12, at The Park School in Norton, described how his friend, who was from a middle-class background, 'turned into a charver (almost)', and they fell out as a consequence. Similarly, Jill Smith, a mother in Norton, described how her daughter's friend had been 'corrupted':

> Um, I think Jane has a friend who's been a charver, who's now come out of it. [. . .] She kind of, you know, went off the rails, but she's now back on the rails but living with the consequences of some of her GCSE choices.

Again we can see a link here in her talk between subcultural groups and valuing of education. Tricia Simpson, a mother in London, revealed a reflexive look at white middle-class fear that their children might be corrupted by white, working-class children, or chavs:

> I think the middle classes tend to stick together and they get on in school circumstances, but they don't outside, so I think worries that middle-class parents have that somehow their children will be sucked into . . . I think some do, I know one or two who have, but, you know . . . [*Interviewer*: 'Sucked into?']. Maybe taken on lifestyles which – become chavs, as Millie would say. Chavvy lifestyle. One of my friends has had children who both drifted down that route. I don't know why. I think they were rebelling against their parents really.

Conclusions

In this article we have discussed the way in which a sample of white, middle-class young people, using English urban state comprehensive schools, construct their working-class 'Other'. We have argued that class is rarely spoken about explicitly but is present in coded terms. We have shown how the different subcultural groupings in certain urban schools have a relationship to raced and classed identities, and how this differs in schools in the three different cities in our research. We have argued that the different ethnic compositions of different cities and schools in those cities result in differing levels of anxiety or threat, and hence denigration of the white working classes. Focusing on constructions of the chav and charver in these young people's talk, we have shown how chavs or charvers are constructed as aesthetically, performatively, and morally different, in opposition to the normative middle-class subject. In this context, chav comes to represent everything about whiteness that the middle classes are not. Through discourses of the chav, we have also explored how class difference is circulated in middle-class discussions around the valuing of education, where distinct divisions in school often fall between those who value education and those who do not, and chavs are the epitome of those who do not. Bourdieu (1984) argues that taste is defined by those who have the power to make their judgements legitimate, and we argue that the white middle classes have more power to place these labels, and define themselves outside this. We show how some of the young people suggest that chav identity is not related to social class and that it is possible to move in and out of this identity, being more or less of charver, or choosing certain aspects of the identity. However, we argue that this perspective not only negates the fact that some people have more power to 'choose' (and to reject) this identity and hence this label, but also shifts responsibility for the consequences of these labels onto individuals who have supposedly 'chosen' this path.

While it is difficult to argue that chav identity maps exactly onto all white, working-class groups (and this is also something the young people in our research refute), we argue that white, middle-class discourses essentialize the white working classes as embodied in the pathologized image of the chav, in which they become 'massified' in the 'middle class imaginary' (Lawler 2005). Skeggs argues that 'class formation is dynamic, produced through conflict and fought out at the level of the symbolic' (2004, p. 5), and that analysis of class should aim to capture the ambiguity produced through struggle and fuzzy boundaries, rather than to fix it in place in order to measure and know it. Chav may not be articulated as classed but this can be described as 'euphemistic transference' (Bromley 2000): the output can be seen to be about class by the forms and perspectives it takes, and the relations it establishes between groups (2004, p. 5). We argue that the way in which the chav is constructed by the white middle classes in our sample, as antithetical to educational success, is classed in its consequences.

Acknowledgements

This paper is drawing on an ESRC-funded research project on Identities, Educational Choice and the White Urban Middle Classes (Award reference RES-148-25-0023), led by Diane Reay, Gill Crozier and David James with Fiona Jamieson and Phoebe Beedell, in addition to the named authors. We would like to thank the rest of the project team for their support and valuable feedback on earlier drafts of this paper. We would also like to thank Kim Allen and Carole Leathwood for their comments on earlier versions.

Notes

1. Identities, Educational Choice and the White Urban Middle Classes (Award reference RES-148-25-0023), led by Diane Reay, Gill Crozier and David James.
2. A comprehensive school is a state-funded secondary school for children from the age of 11 to at least 16 that does not select children on the basis of academic achievement or aptitude.
3. Research in England has found that the top-performing state schools, which include grammar schools (schools with academic selection), other selective state schools (such as church-affiliated schools) and top-performing comprehensive schools feature below-average numbers of children receiving free school meals (used as a proxy for poverty). Children are also more ethnically segregated in their school than in their neighborhood, and more so in densely populated urban areas. Essentially, low-performing state schools contain higher numbers of working-class and minority ethnic children. (See Sutton Trust 2006, Jesson 2008, Burgess *et al.* 2005). Research also shows that independent schools are becoming more popular (IPSOS-MORI 2008).
4. After careful deliberation, the research team decided to anonymize the northern city and the south-west city, to protect the identities of the schools (and hence the participating families) in these cities. It was felt that simply changing the names of the schools would not be enough to render them anonymous. London, we felt was impossible to anonymize, but also less necessary – the sheer numbers of secondary schools in London makes it difficult to identify them once anonymized.
5. We accessed the families through a variety of methods including an article in *The Guardian* newspaper, advertisements in specific sites in gentrified areas of the cities, contacts with urban schools and some snowballing. Parents were told that the research was about the 'white middle classes' and asked to confirm whether they identified as this in order to participate, but we also collected data on parents' occupations and educational backgrounds.
6. There is a long and substantial history of literature in the sociology of education on working-class 'under-achievement' in secondary education in the UK and hostility between working-class and middle-class young people in schools – but this detailed discussion is beyond the scope of this paper (in addition to Willis (1977), notable contributions include Ford (1969), Brown (1987), and Hoggart (1998[1957].))

References

Allen, K., 2008. Young women and the performing arts: creative education, New Labour and the remaking of the young female self. Unpublished PhD thesis. London: Goldsmiths College, University of London.

Archer, L. and Francis, B., 2006. Challenging classes?: exploring the role of social class within the identities and achievement of British Chinese pupils. *Sociology*, 40 (1), 29–49.

Archer, L., Hollingworth, S., and Halsall, A., 2007. University's not for me – I'm a Nike person: urban, working class young people's negotiations of style, identity and educational engagement. *Sociology*, 4 (2), 219–237.

Ball, S.J., 2003. *Class strategies and the education market: the middle classes and social advantage.* London: Routledge Falmer.

Ball, S.J., Maguire, M., and Macrae, S., 2000. *Choice, pathways and transitions post-16: new youth, new economies in the global city.* London: Routledge Falmer.

Bourdieu, P., 1984. *Distinction.* London: Routledge.

Brown, P., 1987. *Schooling ordinary kids: inequality, unemployment and the new vocationalism.* London and New York: Tavistock Publications.

Burgess, S., Wilson, D., and Lupton, R., 2005. Parallel lives? Ethnic segregation in schools and neighbourhoods. *In*: CASE, ed. *CASE papers.* London: CASE.

Butler, T. and Robson, G., 2003. *London calling: the middle classes and the re-making of inner London.* Oxford: Berg.

Byrne, B., 2006. In search of a 'good mix'. 'Race', class, gender and practices of mothering. *Sociology*, 40 (6), 1001–1017.
Crozier, G., Reay, D., James, D., Jamieson, F., Beedell, P., Hollingworth, S., and Williams, K., 2008. White middle class parents, identities, educational choice and the urban comprehensive school: dilemmas, ambivalence and moral ambiguity. *British journal of sociology of education*, 29 (3), 261–272.
Ford, J., 1969. *Social class and the comprehensive school*. London: Routledge and Kegan Paul.
Foucault, M., 1979. *The history of sexuality*. Vol. 1. *An introduction*. London: Penguin.
Furlong, A. and Cartmel, F., 1997. *Young people and social change: individualisation and risk in late modernity*. Buckingham: Open University Press.
Haylett, C., 2001. Illegitimate subjects?: abject whites, neo-liberal modernisation and middle class multiculturalism. *Environment and planning D: society and space*, 19 (3), 351–370.
Hayward, K. and Yar, M., 2006. The chav phenomenon: consumption, media and the construction of a new underclass. *Crime, media, culture*, 2 (1), 9–28.
Hoggart, R., 1998 [1957]. *The uses of literacy*. New Brunswick, NJ: Transaction.
Holt, M. and Griffin, C., 2005. Students versus locals: young adults' constructions of the working class Other. *British journal of social psychology*, 44, 241–267.
IPSOS-MORI, 2008. Independent schools: survey.
Jesson, D., 2008. Grammar schools in the 21st century and social mobility. *BERA research intelligence*, 24–25.
Lawler, S., 2005. Disgusted subjects: the making of middle class identities. *Sociological review*, 53 (3), 429–446.
MacDonald, R., Shildrick, T., Webster, C., and Simpson, D., 2005. Growing up in poor neighbourhoods: the significance of class and place in the extended transitions of 'socially excluded' young adults. *Sociology*, 39 (5), 873–892.
May, J., 1996. Globalization and the politics of place: place and identity in an inner London neighbourhood. *Transactions of the Institute of British Geographers*, NS 21, 194–215.
McCulloch, K., Stewart, A., and Lowegreen, N., 2006. "We just hang out together': youth cultures and social class. *Journal of youth studies*, 9 (5), 539–556.
McDowell, L., 2006. Reconfigurations of gender and class relations. *Antipode*, 38 (4), 825–850.
Miles, S., 2000. *Youth lifestyles in a changing world*. Buckingham: Open University Press.
Nayak, A., 2006. Displaced masculinities: chavs, youth and class in the post-industrial city. *Sociology*, 40 (5), 813–831.
Office for National Statistics, 2005. *Focus on social inequalities*, 2005 edn. London: The Stationery Office.
Raisborough, J. and Adams, M., 2008. Mockery and morality in popular cultural representations of the white working class. *Sociological research online* 13 (6) http://www.socresonline.org.uk/13/6/2.html.
Reay, D., 2004. Exclusivity, exclusion and social class in urban educational markets in the UK. *Urban education*, 39 (5), 537–560.
Reay, D., 2006. The zombie stalking English schools: social class and educational inequality. *British journal of educational studies*, 54 (3), 288–307.
Reay, D., Hollingworth, S., Williams, K., Crozier, G., Jamieson, F., James, D., and Phoebe, B., 2007. A darker shade of pale?: whiteness, the middle classes and multi-ethnic inner city schooling. *Sociology*, 41 (6), 1041–1060.
Redhead, S., 1990. *The end-of-the-century party: youth and pop toward 2000*. Manchester: Manchester University Press.
Rose, N., 1996. Identity, genealogy and history. *In*: S. Hall and P. Du Gay, eds. *Questions of cultural identity*. London: Sage, 128–151.
Sayer, A., 2005a. Class, moral worth and recognition. *Sociology*, 39 (5), 947–964.
Sayer, A., 2005b. *The moral significance of class*. Cambridge: Cambridge University Press.
Sennett, R. and Cobb, J., 1972. *The hidden injuries of class*. Cambridge: Cambridge University Press.
Shildrick, T. and MacDonald, R., 2006. In defence of subculture: young people, leisure and social divisions. *Journal of youth studies*, 9 (2), 125–140.
Skeggs, B., 2004. *Class, self, culture*. London and New York: Routledge.

Skeggs, B., 2005. The making of class through visualising moral subject formation. *Sociology*, 39 (5), 965–982.
Skeggs, B., Wood, H., and Thumin, N., 2007. Making class through moral extension on reality TV. *http://www8.umu.se/medfak/cgf/bev%20warwick%20with%20edits%20_2_.pdf.*
Southerton, D., 2002. Boundaries of 'us' and 'them': class, mobility and identification in a new town. *Sociology*, 36 (1), 171–193.
Sutton Trust, 2006. The social composition of top comprehensive schools – rates of eligibility for free school meals at the 200 highest performing comprehensives. Sutton Trust.
Thorne, B., 1993. *Gender play: girls and boys in school.* Buckinghamshire: Open University Press.
Thornton, S., 1995. *Club cultures: music media and subcultural capital.* Cambridge: Polity Press.
Tyler, I., 2006. Chav scum: the filthy politics of social class in contemporary Britain. *M/C journal*, 9(5). Available from: http://journal.media-culture.org.au/0610/09-tyler.php [Accessed 14 July 2009].
Tyler, I., 2008. 'Chav mum, chav scum': class disgust in contemporary Britain. *Feminist media studies*, 8 (1), 17–34.
Tyler, I. and Bennett, B., forthcoming. Celebrity chav: fame, femininity and social class. *European journal of cultural studies.*
Ward, C., 1990 [1978]. *The child in the city*, New Edition. London: Bedford Square Press.
Wetherell, M. and Potter, J., 1992. *Mapping the language of racism: discourse and the legitimation of exploitation.* Hemel Hempstead: Harvester Wheatsheaf.
Whitty, G., 2001. Education, social class and social exclusion. *Journal of education policy*, 16 (4), 287–295.
Willis, P., 1977. *Learning to labour: why working class kids get working class jobs.* Farnborough: Saxon House.

Who needs enemies with friends like these? The importance of place for young people living in known gang areas

Robert Ralphs, Juanjo Medina and Judith Aldridge

School of Law, University of Manchester, Oxford Road, Manchester, UK

Despite a growing concern about gangs in Britain, academic research that focuses on gangs remains scarce. Drawing on data from the ESRC-funded ethnographic research YOGEC (Youth Gangs in an English City) project, this paper explores the negotiation of space and place by young people living in inner-city areas affected by gangs. Using a combination of fieldwork observations and focus group and interview data, this paper charts the experiences of non-gang-involved young people living in known gang areas. These young people's restricted use of space, arising as a result of gang rivalries and the policing of inner-city areas, results in exclusion, marginalization and victimization. We illustrate how young people are identified as 'high risk', and how they continually negotiate a range of risks bound up with the territory that they inhabit and subsequent spatial boundaries that are formed. In doing so, we provide an understanding of the lives of young people who reside in places and spaces inhabited by gangs.

Introduction

This paper explores the experiences of young people who live in places labelled as 'gang areas' and who therefore are subject to surveillance and interventions by authorities as a result. It seeks to highlight the way that increasing official use of gang terminology impacts on the lives of non-gang-involved young people in their negotiations of the spaces where they live, in ways that are equally as (or more) damaging than peer-based negotiations of space (see Kintrea *et al.* 2008). We also focus on the impact that gangs have on non-gang-involved young people. We illustrate how young people in Britain who reside in places that are recognized as having gang and related firearm problems are restricted in their use of space in ways that go beyond more general accounts of youth, space and territory (Hall *et al.* 1999, Cahill 2000, MacDonald *et al.* 2005, Kintrea *et al.* 2008). We begin with a brief overview of recent British developments of the use of gang terminology among the police, community agencies, and young people themselves; within government policy; and among academic researchers.

British gangs: media hype, public fears and official responses

Young people, particularly, young, working-class males, have long been the source of public fears and the target of the press (Cohen 1972). However, in recent years,

Britain has been 'gripped by gang fever' (Hallsworth and Young, 2004, p. 12); the latest British 'folk devils' are undoubtedly youth gangs. Recent news headlines have included: '500,000 hoodies in gangs' (*The Sun* 2006), 'The trials of living with the feral youths' (*Guardian* 2005) and 'Gun crime growing like cancer' (BBC 2003), as gun and knife crime becomes increasingly intertwined with fears of a growing British 'gang problem'.

In the absence of much recent research with a direct focus on British gangs, government, local authorities and the public are left to rely on these media accounts that 'gang culture' is endemic in our cities and that these gangs resemble popular portrayals of gangs in the USA. This relentless media focus on gangs, alongside the violent deaths of several school-aged young people, has increased the public call for a political response. In February 2007, former Prime Minister Tony Blair presided over Britain's first 'gun crime summit'. This was swiftly followed with the formation of the Home Office's Tackling Gangs Action Programme (TGAP) to identify good practice in dealing with gangs and gun crime. This has resulted in the toolkit: '*Tackling gangs: practical guide for local authorities, Crime Disorder and Reduction Partnerships (CDRPS) and other local partners*' (Home Office 2008) and a government guidance leaflet for parents on how to detect children's involvement in gangs. In Britain, academics and public bodies such as the Youth Justice Board rightly warn against the dangers of a too liberal use of gang labels; yet, the term 'gang' has become entrenched in both national and local crime and disorder strategies (e.g. Home Office 2008). Police forces and local authorities are increasingly drawing on US interventions by importing models developed in Los Angeles and Boston of dedicated firearm/gang units and multi-agency gang intervention teams, now firmly established within some British cities (Bullock and Tilley 2008, Home Office 2008).

The recent British government and local authority responses outlined here to the ostensibly increased threat posed by youth gangs – and their alleged increased use of firearms – can be understood within the theoretical discourses of risk. Many commentators have argued that we live in a society transfixed with risk (Beck 1992, Garland 2001). As a society, the management of risk is paramount to our ontological security (Giddens 1991). Reactionary policies around youth gangs can in part counter the public's fear (Garland 2001). The heightened level of risk deemed to result from youth gangs – primarily through the growing concern that they are increasingly using firearms – is new in a British context. This link between 'gangs' and guns has elevated established concerns of youth as 'troublesome' and 'folk devils' (Cohen 1972) to their being viewed as 'ruthless assassins' and 'high risk'. This is particularly the case for young people residing in 'gang areas', who are subject to labels and methods of 'risk management' that are damaging in many ways. Indeed, we must be mindful not to label our young people (Lemert 1951, Becker 1963). In 2007, prior to resigning as Chair of England and Wales Youth Justice Board, Professor Rod Morgan warned that we risk demonizing a whole generation, by labelling young people as 'thugs in hooded tops' and 'gang members' (Youth Justice Board 2007).

Policing gangs and young people: the story so far

While the formation of dedicated firearm/gang units by police in Britain is a relatively new phenomenon, gang units have existed for two decades in the USA.

During this time, many US researchers have questioned, in particular, the quality of gang-related intelligence and derived gang-members databases. Katz and Webb (2006) provide a useful and comprehensive overview. Some have suggested that police officials have arbitrarily classified individuals as gang members (Parachini and Crew 1996, cited in Katz *et al.* 2000). Others have noted how 'hearsay information' about gang affiliation is incorporated into intelligence systems (Burrell 1990, Spergel 1995), resulting in individuals being unfairly labelled gang members solely as a consequence of the neighbourhood where they live, their relationship with a known gang member, or their style of dress (Hagedorn 1990, Chesney-Lind *et al.* 1994). Others are even more scathing: in their study of gangs in Las Vegas, McCorkle and Miethe (1998) concluded that the 'gang problem' could be attributed to a moral panic constructed by the police department to obtain resources and regain legitimacy within the community. On the other hand, there are researchers who have argued that 'gang information systems may be more helpful to police than first believed' and that they correctly identify criminally active individuals (Katz *et al.*, 2000, p. 432). In Britain, these controversial US gang interventions have slipped unquestioned into mainstream policy and practice. It is probable that adopting a similar model of US gang interventions and surveillance will result in similar gang labelling practices. Indeed, in tracking the development of a Manchester-based gang intervention programme that was based on the Boston Gun Project, Bullock and Tilley (2008, p. 38) have noted 'unresolved concerns about the risks of labelling and stereotyping young people', as well as poorly evidenced 'gang membership'.

Several studies have highlighted how the police construct populations of 'permanent suspects' based on socio-economic status as much as on serious and persistent offending. These studies also note how 'street life' places young people at greater risk of adversarial contact with authority (Aye-Maung 1995, Flood-Page *et al.* 2000, McAra and McVie 2005). There is a substantial body of literature that discusses how police 'working rules' are used to construct a suspect population (McConville *et al.* 1991, 1997, Smith 1991, Reiner 1997, Quinton *et al.* 2000). These informal rules, based on police culture, are said to impact differently according to a range of demographics. One such important demographic, as we will discuss in this paper, is area of residence. The new policing of gangs and gang members, through the use of dedicated gang units with a remit to target youth gangs in particular areas, has the potential to intensify police attention on young people who have the misfortune to reside in known gang areas.

The links between gangs and gun crime is also significant for the policing of young people in known gang areas. There is a long history in Britain in relation to problematic police stop-and-search practices, particularly in relation to ethnic minorities (see Scarman 1981, Bowling and Phillips 2002, Sharp and Atherton 2007). Yet, despite the introduction of the Police and Criminal Evidence Act (PACE 1984) and subsequent amendments to the recording requirements for all stops – whether a search ensues or not (Home Office 2004) – due process is clouded by Section 60 of the Criminal Justice and Public Order Act 1994. Section 60, once authorized by an inspector (typically for a 24-hour period), allows officers to stop and search any individual within a defined area without 'reasonable suspicion' when it is anticipated that serious violence may occur or that offensive weapons such as firearms may be carried.[1] The constant threat of gun crime in known gang areas, coupled with increased police surveillance by dedicated firearm and gang units, intensifies police attention on young people living in these areas and results in more vulnerability to excessive stop and search.

The enduring significance of class and place in youth experiences

In recent decades, it has been suggested that social class is of diminishing significance, as globalization has led to a more risk-based society (Beck 1992). Social theorists have similarly downplayed the importance of place, noting that growing geographical mobility has resulted in everyday experiences becoming increasingly disembedded from physical location (Calhoun 1991, Giddens 1991). In specific relation to youth studies, Blackman (2005) has been critical of postmodern, post-subcultural theory that places greater emphasis on agency and the individual at the expense of critical discussion of the structures and institutions that exist and continue to marginalize some sections of young people. He notes the lack of critical application to young people's social, economic and cultural realities. It is important that youth research seeks to address this omission, as Shildrick and MacDonald (2006, p. 126) argue: 'A proper, holistic understanding of youth *requires* a closer appreciation of the ways in which young people's leisure and cultural lives intersect with wider aspects of their biographies.' In these critiques of post-subcultural studies, both Blackman (2005) and Shildrick and MacDonald (2006) have pointed to the tendency to empirically ignore the lives and identities of less advantaged young people, while theoretically underplaying the potential significance of class and other social inequalities.[2]

In contrast, MacDonald *et al.* (2005) have stressed the continuing importance of class and place for young people. Kintrea *et al.* (2008) reached a similar conclusion in their study of territoriality and territorial conflict in six British cities, stating that all the areas they encountered with 'territorial conflict' were areas containing multiple disadvantage. Significantly, they found this type of conflict to be much less evident in the more advantaged areas of each city. Kintrea and colleagues also suggest that the limitations that ensue as a result of young people's restricted spatial mobility actually inhibit transitions to adult life, as, for example, by restricting access to education. The lives of the young people presented in these recent British studies are highly bound up with their social class and the places they lived. Youth gangs similarly challenge the notion that class and place are not important in understanding young people's lives. Gang research has long associated gangs with the most deprived areas in inner cities (Thrasher 1927, Shaw and McKay 1942, Cohen 1955, Miller 1958, Cloward and Ohlin 1960, Parker 1974). Hagedorn (1988) uses an 'urban underclass' framework while Venkatesh (1997, p. 82) similarly notes how street gangs, together with teenage pregnancy and welfare state dependency, have become a 'signature attribute of ghetto life'. More recently, Vigil (2002) refers to 'multiple marginality' in his explanation of the existence of gangs across a range of diverse communities.

As with class, the links between gangs and space are important. Tita *et al.* (2005) have noted that not only are gangs spatially concentrated among disadvantaged neighbourhoods, but also, within this, they occupy what they term 'gang set space'. These are geographically defined areas within a neighbourhood where gang members 'hang out'. Klein (1995, p. 18) refers to these areas where gangs hang out as 'the life space of the gang'.

Kintrea *et al.* (2008) are the latest to note the bounded use of space by young people, due to (potential) conflict with other peers. For the most part, Kintrea *et al.* (2008) steer clear of using the term 'gang', instead bypassing the problems of gang definitions by focusing on 'territoriality'. Hence, they take the well-trodden path in British academia of avoiding a direct focus on the 'gang'.[3] In contrast, the focus here is firmly on 'gangs' and the implications of gang labels for places and the young people who live there. We do not refer here to 'gangs' unproblematically. Indeed, what follows is a highly critical account of the dangers and impact on young people's lives that the over-liberal use of the terms 'gang member' and 'gang associate' can entail. This additional focus on official responses to 'youth gangs' highlights a further dimension to young people's negotiations of space and place that goes beyond peer conflict.

This paper presents the experiences of non-gang-involved young people who live in areas of a city where gangs and gun crime are firmly established. We explore how the risks associated with gangs and gun crime lead young people wrongly identified as gang members or associates to develop coping strategies and how policy-level responses impact negatively on them, and in turn, on their identity, future aspirations and transitions to adulthood. As will be illustrated, in known gang areas the gang labels and treatment that follow form a central part of young people's experiences.

Methods

The findings presented in this paper are based upon the ESRC-funded YOGEC (Youth Gangs in an English City) ethnographic study, which involved 26 months of participant observation, nine focus groups and 107 formal interviews. Time was spent hanging around and socializing with gang members, their associates, ex-gang members and other young people in 'gang' communities. Fieldwork also included attendance at community events, volunteering in youth centres frequented by gang- and non-gang-involved young people, and involvement in community groups concerned with gang violence. The data analysed here draw extensively on two focus group interviews with non-gang youth, interviews with 'gang associates' and with senior police officers, and fieldwork observations of young people who live in known gang areas.

The research took place in an English city, and to maintain its anonymity it is referred to here as 'Research City'. This brief summary of the methods used glosses over many challenges and adaptations to the original research outline. For a more detailed discussion of the methodology and the rationale for the decision not to disclose the name of the city, see Aldridge *et al.* (2008). The research covered six 'gang' areas of the city. The focus in this paper is on one area of the city where gangs were most entrenched, referred to here as *Inner West*. This area encompassed some of the most ethnically diverse and disadvantaged areas of the city and had a gang problem that was widely recognized by the police, young people, the local communities, the city council, and a range of statutory and voluntary sector organizations. When discussing 'gangs' here, our starting point for a working definition in our research was the Eurogang definition: 'Any durable street orientated youth group whose involvement in illegal activity is part of their group identity.'[4] Although not explicit in this definition, the use of firearms was an important defining feature of gangs for city authorities. Some of the more established gangs associated with this area have been in existence for up to 20 years. They have been viewed as responsible for a series of fatal shootings and serious woundings of predominantly young males (aged 14 to 25). During the fieldwork, six young males from this area were fatally shot and many more shot at and injured.

Results

Everyone's a target: restrictions on the use of public space as a consequence of fear and gang victimization

Living in known gang areas significantly limited the use of space for the non-gang young people in our research. When discussing the boundaries of the areas where they felt safe, several young people in one focus group described the space between two local fast-food takeaways – a mere 500 metres apart. When asked what they feared, these non-gang young people would typically cite the risk of street robbery and/or assault by gangs from rival areas and, in common with known gang members, they ultimately feared being shot. It was common for these young people to discuss the problems they experienced when venturing into an area whose gangs have established rivalries with gangs in their area. When young people encountered others from rival gang areas, typically they would be asked: 'Who you down with?' and some young people reported that their mobile phone contact lists were searched through with repercussions possible depending on whom they were found to associate with. These confrontations occurred on public transport and in the city centre, shopping centres, and entertainment venues, as well as in rival gang areas. The fear of victimization that resulted restricted the mobility of these non-gang young people. The problems they encountered are discussed by participants in this focus group:

> Yeah, if you go out of your own area, if you're dressed like some hot boy[5] and that, black clothing and that, then people will attack you and that and they ask you questions. [IWFG41: 16-year-old, white male]

> We can't go to Main Road. [. . .] We go to Main Road, yeah, and straight away, 'Yeah, there's a Upperside man, let's get him.' [IWFG11: 15-year-old, white male]

The risk of being a victim of gun crime intensified young people's fears of venturing into rival gang areas:

> I've got a brother, I fret when he leaves the estate. You understand where I'm coming from? Because he's going out to people that are not from around here, and might not like people off this estate. Do you understand where I'm coming from? And it makes you trapped; it makes you feel trapped anyway. Because you think, 'Well if I move out, I'm gonna have to move way out.' Because there are certain places, because your list or whatever is so long, there is gang members, and you might get to know them. And like there's people, you might have known them before they were gang members, and know them just as that person. And then you know all those people over there who want to kill him, you know what I mean, so you're not gonna go over there. But you've got to go over there to see your friends. [*Interviewer*: Because they might associate you with them, yeah?] And I'm not a gang member, but I might have friends. You get where I'm coming from? So therefore it would make me wary going in certain places. [IWFG42: 18-year-old, white female]

The fear of becoming embroiled in violent encounters led many young people to stay within particular areas within their neighbourhoods. However, as we discuss below, remaining within the confines of these areas did not offer complete protection either, as it could also lead to unwanted attention from both rival gangs and the police.

While gangs may be associated with an entire neighbourhood or housing estate, 'set space' refers to the specific streets, spaces and buildings where gang members are known to congregate (Tita *et al.* 2005). In Research City, these set spaces were evident and of central importance in the process of labelling young people as gang members. Young people who attended certain youth and community buildings where gangs were known to go or who resided in these set spaces became labelled as gang members or gang associates by rival gangs – despite a lack of self-identification or criminality (two factors common to many gang definitions), as this white, male police intelligence officer discusses:

> West Park, I would say from experience, is the heart of Lowerside territory. Now rightly or wrongly, any male seen in that area, who frequents that area, would be regarded by opposing factions as being a gang member and that is very sad, but unfortunately that's how it's progressed. Likewise anyone on Long Lane, Upperside Gang, bang, they're going to be tarred with that brush, whether they've got allegiance and you know it's got to that extreme. [KI12]

Young people had to navigate carefully the known gang places and spaces within their neighbourhoods. Gang set spaces became targets for rival gang attacks, with instances of drive-by shootings and one instance during fieldwork of a rival gang entering community buildings in balaclavas. These kinds of events resulted in local young people refusing to occupy these spaces, understandably deeming them 'unsafe'. This resulted in well-resourced, purpose-built facilities for young people remaining empty and underused. Many of the young people who lived close to youth facilities told us how they did not frequent them due to fear of harassment or even drive-by shootings from rival gangs. This view is summed up here by this young man:

> There are loads of people that ain't gang members that get shot. [. . .] 'We've seen you speaking to so-and-so so we're coming for you.' [. . .] I think everyone's a target; every young person in the area is a target really, if you're in the wrong place at the wrong time. [IWGA6: 15-year-old, black male]

This view is echoed here:

> They don't care who you are. As long as you're on that estate they'll just – they'll just shoot at anything. It could be even your little brother. There's been people playing on bouncy castles, and people driving by and shooting. The bouncy castle's getting popped and that. [IWFG41: 16-year-old, white male]

Young people living in these areas therefore perceived themselves to be at risk of serious violent attacks simply by being in the wrong place. Residing in these areas also had consequences in terms of how the police would view and subsequently police young people.

'By the company that he keeps': the significance of place for police applications of gang labels

Fearful of venturing into areas with gangs in rivalry to their own areas, non-gang young people would limit themselves to their local streets and places where they felt safer. This invariably brought them into contact with suspected gang members from their own areas. Their occupation of these spaces once more proved important in relation to police responses to them. The police employed similar strategies to those of rival gangs when evaluating whether somebody was a gang member, most often based on being seen in the company of known gang members. The way young people were labelled as 'gang members' or 'gang associates' is illustrated here by a police officer with over a decade of experience of working on gang-related crime in this part of the city:

> It's difficult to quantify gang members. I mean certainly there's like, you know, three or more engaged in criminal activity blah, blah, blah and all this business, and I always turn round and say, 'OK, if somebody says to me, "Is Joe Bloggs a gang member?" And I will obviously look at what we know about him and say, 'Well, if he's been stop-checked once or twice with a known gang member, he's on the periphery.' But he's getting stop-checked regular, then you've got to say, 'Well, look, by the company that he keeps we believe that he's a gang member.' [KI12]

Consistent with previous accounts of police practice and 'working rules' (see McConville *et al.* 1991, McAra and McVie 2005), young people attracted police attention as a result of keeping the wrong company rather than as a result of involvement in criminal activity. Indeed, being seen in the company of 'known' gang members was crucial to the police application of the gang label in Research City. In the absence of a clear official definition of what constitutes a 'gang member' in practice, association was both a necessary and sufficient condition for the application of the label, and despite a strong association in Research City between gangs and serious crime, criminal engagement was not a necessary official defining feature of gang membership for the police, let alone co-offending with known gang members. For those living or socializing in gang set spaces, it is inevitable that they will come into contact with gang members. Moreover, as a strategy of self-defence, to befriend 'the gang' would seem logical. The non-gang young people we spoke to perceived behaving in a superficially friendly manner to gang members they knew (for example, greeting them in the street) was an effective strategy to avoid being victimized by them. Indeed, many young people who knew and had grown up with gang members, including siblings, often expressed negative views of gangs and the related activities gang members engaged in, especially serious violence and other forms of criminality. However, young people living in these areas were regularly stop-checked by police; the suspicion of gang involvement would result if they were in the company of those police considered to be 'known' gang members. Because police designate gang affiliation on the basis of being seen with 'known' gang members, it is inevitable that these observations will result in false positives.

Lemert (1951) and Becker (1963) describe the impact of deviant labels in relation to the potential for secondary deviance and further criminality. What we witnessed in our research was the potential for entire neighbourhoods (especially those living in gang set spaces) of young people to be labelled as 'gang members' or 'gang associates' and to receive high levels of police attention as a consequence of being born and raised in estates and streets with established gang associations. This young man describes being considered by the police to be a member of a 40-strong gang:

> I don't even think there really is a gang in Shanklytown. [*Interviewer*: So all the ones like I mentioned to you before, you know, the police have said there's about 40...] 40 Crestside Crew and all that! [laughs] [*Interviewer*: So what would you say?] I would say

> there's about three, innit. ... They aren't in Crestside Crew yeah, 'cause the police have said to me if you're seen speaking to a gang member, if they see you speaking to a gang member, automatically they put you in a gang. [*Interviewer*: So the police have said that to you?] Yeah, so the 40 people that they say, that could just be, they're young people from Crestside, that like, these three gang members I spoke to. And then, like, if you say that I'm in a gang, if they see me speaking to a gang member now, who I speak to must be in a gang too and who they speak to. It's daft really. [IWGA8: 16-year-old, black male]

McAra and McVie (2005) have noted a similar cycle of police labelling of young people in Scotland, in which young people with friends known to the police are twice as likely to come into contact with the police, regardless of any criminality. In Research City, the specific association with gangs and gun crime elevates these more general police suspicions to another level. Many of the young people we got to know during the fieldwork became labelled as gang members or gang associates, even where they did not self-define as a gang member, held strongly anti-gang views, and did not engage in criminal activity. Nevertheless, once labelled, they were treated – by police and subsequently by other agencies such as schools – as capable of serious crimes, or as posing potential or actual risks as a result of the label. The following section outlines some of the repercussions of these gang labels.

Police surveillance, raids, stops and searches and other spatial restrictions

Being labelled as a gang member or associate created a greater vulnerability to police attention and surveillance. Armed police raids on family homes in search for firearms were common and brought stigma, stress and feelings of violation to the families involved. Young people living in these areas and labelled as 'gang associates' were often subjected to police checks and exclusion from community events including carnivals and family fun days. We regularly attended these events and witnessed how young people from the youth clubs where we worked were sometimes prevented from entering, and on occasion, overtly filmed by the police. Their access was denied due to apparent gang associations on the grounds of public safety and potential conflict between rival gangs. Again, many of these young people had no criminal history and did not view themselves as gang involved. Likewise, their peers did not see them as gang members, nor did members of the gangs that they were allegedly affiliated to, as we know from conversations and interviews with gang members and associates.

The police adopted a proactive method of harassment of people they identified as 'gang members'. When known gang members were visible on the streets where they live, they had to negotiate unwanted attention from the police as well as from rival gangs, who may target their hangouts with drive-by shootings, as this gang intelligence officer noted:

> If we suddenly see Crestside Crew emerging on Long Lane, bang, get over there, get our uniform lads to absolutely hammer them, harass them, do them for anything they can. So they basically think, 'We've had enough of this', and we can dampen things down [...] but [hanging around on the streets] from our point of view makes them a target. Lowerside lads can drive by, so if we're dispersing them and displacing them, it's diminishing the problem again. [KI16]

Earlier, it was noted how streets and places become known as gang set spaces, and this is clearly evident in this account, as is the risk of drive-by shootings by rival gangs. This police 'harassment' tactic was frequently discussed by the non-gang young people who lived in these areas, as this young man discusses:

> Like when the police say, 'Where are you from?' and you say like, 'Belmont', straight away, 'Have you been in trouble?' 'No.' 'Are you sure?' 'Yeah.' 'Right, let me PNC[6] your ID. Are you sure you've not been in trouble before? I'll check. Have you got any guns on you? Rear[7] always asking you. [IWFG12: 16-year-old, white male]

A focus group with non-gang youth in a rival gang area uncovered similar experiences:

> *IWFG43: 17-year-old, white male*: They judge everyone the same; they judge every person the same, no matter like how you dress and that.
>
> *IWFG42: 18-year-old, white female*: Yeah if you haven't got serial numbers on your shoulder, that's how they go on really, you know.
>
> *IWFG44: 16-year-old, Asian male*: Yeah and if you talk back to them, then they think he's Windham Gang.
>
> *IWFG43: 17-year-old, white male*: If you're dressed in all black, he'll see you as a gang member.

As this discussion indicates, young people viewed this type of unwanted (and in their view unwarranted) police attention and continued stop-checks – both formal and informal – as police harassment. Non-gang young people from these areas recounted being stopped by the police at least weekly, often two or three times per week, and on occasion, two or three times per day. Their experiences are typified in the following focus group discussion:

> [*Interviewer*: So how many times have you been stopped by the police?]
> It just depends. Say if I went to Ashland, yeah, I'd get pulled like twice a day. If you go into Ashland, yeah, they're just pulling you, 'Where are you from? Where are you from?' 'Belmont.' 'Yeah, what are you doing round here? Coming round causing trouble?' [IWFG11: 16-year-old, white male]
>
> [*Interviewer*: So on average, how many times do you get stopped?] Well, the most about three times a week. [IWFG12: 16-year-old, white male]
>
> [*Interviewer*: And what about other people, is that the same for everybody?] No, some are getting picked – like some are getting followed around all day long. [IWFG11: 16-year-old, white male]
>
> Well, about three weeks ago I got stopped and searched every day within like – for about seven days it was, but every day continuously. [IWFG43: 17-year-old, white male]

Previous studies have indicated that the type of repeated negative police contact documented here helps to reinforce young people's hostility to the police (Flood-Page *et al.* 2000, McAra and McVie 2005). These repeated altercations with the police resulted, for the young people in our research, in antagonistic relationships with the police and mistrust of them, as illustrated, for example, by their unwillingness to report crimes against them to the police or to assist the police in their enquiries. Not surprisingly then, many young people held a negative attitude to the police:

[*Interviewer*: So how would you describe your relationship with the police, then?]

IWFG11: 16-year-old, white male: Bastards.

IWFG15: 14-year-old, black male: Sort of like bastards.

IWFG18: 15-year-old, white male: Pests.

IWFG12: 15-year-old, black male: Yeah.

IWFG16: 16-year-old, white male: Like fucking cockroaches.

Several: [laugh]

This hostility shown to the police together with more general mistrust and lack of confidence in the local police force is consistent with recent research from both the USA (Brunson and Miller 2006) and Britain (Sharp and Atherton 2007). It is telling here that non-gang young people, regardless of ethnicity, reported similar experiences and perceptions of the police. However, while the police responded to all young people in these areas as potential gang members, regardless of ethnic origin, ethnicity was important in how police defined areas as 'gang areas' and individuals as 'gang members', as we will discuss in more depth in future publications.

The impact of living in known gang areas: gang labelling and its consequences

Much of the literature on the labelling process (Lemert 1951, Becker 1963) and constructions of 'suspect populations' (McConville *et al.* 1991, Quinton *et al.* 2000) has focused on how these deviant labels and associations can lead to further criminality. Setting aside the question of whether, or the extent to which, the application of labels can lead to actual gang joining,[8] here we describe a range of other consequences of the use of one specific kind of deviant label, the gang label – applied to both individuals and communities.

The labelling of young people as gang members or associates not only affected their experiences and use of public space but also their interactions with authorities. These gang association labels affected their experiences in secondary and further education, their aspirations, and ultimately their transitions to adulthood. To illustrate the magnitude of the consequences gang labels can have for young people, one young man's experience is discussed here as a case study. The problems he encountered including school exclusion, police raids and excessive police monitoring were recounted and experienced by several other young people known to the research team.

Dwain (not his real name), a 16-year-old black male, frequented a youth club where the lead author worked as a volunteer. He aspired to work in the music industry and to study law. He had never been arrested or charged with any offence. He was interviewed because of having several cousins involved in gangs. The youth clubs he frequented were also attended by gang members and he lived on the same street as several known gang members. Consequently, his street and local youth club were classed by police as 'gang set spaces' (Tita *et al.* 2005). He expressed anti-gang attitudes: 'Gang stuff is just daft' and condemned individual gang members: 'There's only a few smart ones that make money. The rest of them are just daft.' Nevertheless, he was considered to be a gang member or associate by the police and subsequently treated as a risk to his school. His response to this was damning: 'If they're telling me that I'm in a gang, they don't know anything.'

Yet, despite his denial and demands made to police to see the intelligence that led to this label, the association remained and resulted in a sequence of highly exclusionary events. During his final year of secondary school, a few months before his final exams, his school was informed by the police that he was a gang member, although they were unable to specify which gang due to insufficient evidence. Although never arrested for any offence or known to be involved in gang conflict in his school, he was temporarily suspended. The police evidence for this association was requested by his family but, at this stage, was not forthcoming.[9] He recalled how his school justified his suspension:

> They were saying to me that if I'm in a gang, that's bringing trouble for the school, 'cause that will bring the gang members to the school and that, after school and that, and kids will get robbed and all that, just talking rubbish. [Interviewer: They're saying that's down to you?] Yeah, that I'm a risk to the school if I'm in a gang and all that.

Being excluded from school was not an isolated occurrence for young people living in these known gang areas. Fortunately, Dwain was eventually able to return to school and sit his exams. The practice of excluding young people from schools highlights the emerging trend of a heightened sense of risk that schools, local authorities and police forces are alert to. At another school, a high-achieving student in his penultimate year, together with two school friends, was permanently excluded after a group of young men had gathered at the school gates and threatened to kill him. This event resulted in the school seeking guidance from local authority and police personnel who work on gang interventions. They labelled him as a 'gang member', as a result of family links to gangs and subsequently, despite being a good student with no previous school warnings or involvement in crime, he was excluded because he posed a 'serious risk to students and staff safety'.[10] It is difficult to find a replacement school when a young person is deemed as posing a 'high risk' to students and staff. In addition, his status as a victim of crime was ignored and his exclusion meant that he was once more victimized.

Exclusionary experiences like the ones illustrated here have wider implications for young people's transitions to employment. Young people in these areas frequently discussed the way that they felt excluded and marginalized because of the area where they lived. Others had fractious relationships with the education system as well as with the police. Non-gang young people discussed how teachers, aware of where they lived, would predict that they would end up a 'drug dealer', a 'gang member' or 'dead'. This may contribute to the low aspirations among young people we encountered in the research. Those who did pursue further education and job training recounted how they were negatively judged once they disclosed where they lived, as this 17-year-old, white male stated:

> Well, I've been like at Westside College, and all these teachers and that, they're all like from Westside [a suburban area], you know, all posh places like that. So when they go, 'Where are you from?' and then like you mention Belmont, they look at you weird, they judge you weird, because they're used to like, you know, the posh areas, being able to walk around the streets and all that. [*Interviewer*: So even when you're out of the area like that and you're in college, you think you get treated...?] If you mention where

you're from, they will judge you, the same as other people would, where you are. [IWFG43: 17-year-old, white male]

These experiences and perceptions had important consequences. During fieldwork, we encountered numerous examples of young people who had given up on seeking employment, long before they had reached the official school-leaving age of 16. Young people would refer to the stigma that their gang-affected area had and how nobody would give them a job once they knew their postcode. Regardless of whether these views hold true, their perceptions, enforced by negative interactions with police and other officials, were enough to make many young people give up trying. As noted earlier, young people (whether gang or non-gang affiliated) living in these known gang areas – gang or non-gang affiliated – experienced a curtailing of their geographical and social movement. This limited mobility consequently restricted their access to services. Hence, not all young people are able to access leisure and other services in the same way and therefore, as Ball *et al.* (2000) observe, the capacity to participate and consume varies among young people in dependence on structural factors, with social class and place clearly relevant here to these young people's experiences (see also Bose 2003, Blackman 2005, Shildrick and MacDonald 2006).

Discussion and conclusions

Our findings confirm the view that the social construction and regulation of public space are further contributing to the social exclusion of marginalized young people (White 1996) and that this has become more of a problem with the development of new regulatory practices and powers (Collins and Kearns 2001). Policy responses to gangs may contribute to these exclusionary processes and lead to social control mechanisms with the characteristics outlined by Stanley Cohen (1979) in his well-known, dystopian essay 'The Punitive City': blurred boundaries between inside and out, guilty and innocent; broadened and increasingly fuzzy definitions of crime; an expanded social control net; and dispersed state social control mechanisms beyond prison (or office) walls.

In the British context, recent academic discussion of gangs has tended to focus on definitions of what a gang is and whether they even exist (see Hallsworth and Young 2004, Young *et al.* 2007, Pitts 2008). The experiences presented here of young people living in known gang areas has clearly demonstrated that a serious problem for many young people who reside in these areas concerns the individual level definition of who is a 'gang member' or 'gang associate'. The accounts from non-gang-involved young people and those who dispute their gang-status labels illustrate that the less discriminate use of these terms by both gang-involved youth and officials has severe implications for the personal safety and exclusion of those who live in known gang areas.

It is commonly understood that the organization of youth gangs is fluid and their membership difficult to identify (Esbensen *et al.* 2001, Sullivan 2005). Yet, the evidence presented here demonstrates that local authorities and police forces often seem to apply the gang label based on association in gang-affected neighbourhoods – that is, observing a young person together with a 'known gang member'. These labels have serious consequences for those born and raised in such areas. We encountered a growing concern within these communities over the use of official gang labels with information of varying quality about individuals suspected of gang activity. Young people with family relationships to gang members, who attended the same schools, youth provisions or set spaces, or who lived on the same streets as gang members were in danger of being considered by police to be gang members themselves, or at least 'gang associated' and subjected to increased surveillance and intervention, regardless of criminal involvement. This resulted in exclusion from community events and, more worryingly, exclusion from the education system.

In areas with established gang associations, it is difficult, if not impossible, for young people to avoid association with gang members. They attended the same local schools, youth and community centres; places of worship; and sports, music and drama groups, and hung out on the same streets. This was particularly the case for those young people who lived in gang set spaces. Hence, when spotted in conversation or stopped and searched by the police, they would often be labelled as 'gang associated' if not as fully fledged 'gang members'. Rival gangs also interpreted these types of interactions with known gang members and sightings in gang set spaces as a sign of gang membership or allegiance. The result, as illustrated here, was as serious as permanent school exclusion, dawn raids by armed police and victimization. The young people who resided in these already marginalized areas were subsequently victims of further marginalization, exclusion and stigmatization, which increased their levels of disaffection and diminished their opportunities.

Place and class were central to these experiences. Young people encountered in these working-class areas associated with gangs were victimized, marginalized and excluded in many ways, as a consequence of this association – regardless of whether they were gang members or not. Historically, it has been widely accepted that gangs emerge under conditions of social exclusion. What these findings have highlighted is that further social exclusion of young people is a by-product of areas becoming firmly associated with gangs. We therefore need to identify strategies for the policing of gangs that are both successful and respectful of civil liberty concerns. With the increasing focus on risk management, the types of practices of some of our most marginalized young people that we have documented are likely not only to persist but also to expand and intensify. This is evident in the current climate of governmental concern around dealing with youth gangs (Home Office 2008) and continued investment and expansion of dedicated police units and other statutory agencies with a remit to target 'youth gangs'. Ironically, this type of persistent policing may well contribute to offending behaviour (McAra and McVie 2005), police mistrust (Sharp and Atherton 2007), poor legal socialization (Fagan and Tyler 2005) and perhaps reinforced gang identities.

The lived reality of the young people we encountered, regardless of their status as 'gang member', 'gang associate' or 'non-gang', was one of marginalization and exclusion. This is in contrast to the picture painted in the British media of fearless young people marauding through our cities. They are instead highly *fearful*. Already living in deprived neighbourhoods, they are further excluded and victimized through association with gangs. MacDonald *et al.* (2005, p. 873) note how 'Locally embedded social networks become part of the process whereby poverty and class inequalities are reproduced.' In this instance, youth gangs can be seen as one form of social network that serves to reproduce inequalities. The interactions with authorities and other young people may further bolster 'gang culture'.

In line with both Kintrea *et al.* (2008) and Marshall *et al.* (2004), this paper has highlighted young people's fears of leaving the streets and estates where they live due to perceived threats of gangs from surrounding areas. For young people living in the most disadvantaged areas, this limited mobility can further reinforce their social exclusion and limit their access to services. As Kintrea *et al.* (2008, p. 14) note, 'It is not just the fact of the negative impacts of territorial behaviour that appears to be the issue for young people, but also that they occur at a crucial stage in their lives.' In this respect, their subsequent transitions to adulthood are affected by these social and physical restrictions.

Inner-city neighbourhood reputations can be extremely negative (e.g. Fraser 1996). In our research, we adopted the strategy of not disclosing publicly the neighbourhoods – even the city – in which our research was conducted, at least in part to avoid further stigmatizing what we anticipated would be communities already feeling stigmatized by 'gang' reputations and by other markers of inner-city deprivation. We assess this strategy as vindicated in part by the results reported in this paper. We have shown that the gang label is indeed a dangerous one – and not just for young people involved in gangs but also for the young people living in gang-affected areas who are wrongly assumed to be gang members by the police and rival gangs based on their use of place and space, as well as more broadly for non-gang young people who are often victimized and stigmatized as they carry with them the reputations of having come from gang-affected neighbourhoods.

Acknowledgements

The research for this paper was funded by the ESRC (RES-000-23-0615), and entitled 'Youth Gangs in an English City'.

Notes

1. Section 60 was typically used in the days that followed a shooting incident. The use of Section 60 was also common at events such as carnivals or other community and musical events where the police anticipated attendance by gang members.
2. Shildrick and MacDonald (2006, p. 129) note the paradox that, in contrast to the popular media focus on young, working-class 'hoodies, 'gangs' and general anti-social behaviour, discussed above, in much of the contemporary academic studies on youth and leisure, the cultural identities and practices of working-class youth – especially the most marginalized and disadvantaged sections – rarely feature.
3. This reluctance to use gang terminology in Britain dates back almost half a century (see Downes 1966), and the term remains highly contested to the present day (see also Young *et al.* 2007).
4. The Eurogang Network was formed with the remit of agreeing consistent definition, questions and methodologies to allow comparative international gang research. For more information see its website at: http://www.umsl.edu/~ccj/eurogang/euroganghome.htm.
5. The term 'hot boy' was used locally by young people to describe young males who were frequently talked about due to what they were involved in. This could mean they were regularly stopped by the police, or wanted/attacked by rival gangs, or known to carry a weapon such as a firearm. The term was also more generically used to refer to somebody who dressed and acted like a stereotypical gang member. Its origins may lie in the 1999 film *Hot Boyz* (also known as *Gang Law*), a US gangster movie starring the rap artist Snoop Dog.
6. 'PNC' refers here to the Police National Computer. When the police stop a member of the public, this national computer system is used to check for any additional information such

as outstanding warrants for arrest or previous convictions, or to confirm that the information provided is consistent.

7. 'Rear' or more typically, 'rear, rear, rear' was often used in conversation by many people when they were recounting an event or conversation in the same way that 'etc., etc.' or 'and so on' are more commonly used.
8. The possible reasons why young people become involved in gangs will be discussed in future publications with a focus on onset of gang involvement/membership.
9. It took a subsequent official police complaint against his treatment and labelling as a gang member to ascertain the police intelligence that led to this label. It emerged that on a couple of occasions when he had been routinely stopped by the police in his neighbourhood (a regular occurrence for him and other young people in his area), he was in the company of suspected gang members or 'naughty lads', as one officer put it.
10. Ironically, a consistent theme that emerged through discussion and interviews with gang members was how the education system failed them. Leaving school was identified as a 'critical moment' for either the onset of gang involvement or more sustained gang and offending involvement.

References

Aldridge, J., Medina, J., and Ralphs, R., 2008. Dangers and problems of doing 'gang' research. *In*: F. van Gemert, D. Peterson and I. Lien, eds. *Street gangs, migration and ethnicity.* Cullompton: Willan Publishing, 31–46.

Aye-Maung, N., 1995. *Young people, victimisation and the police: British crime survey findings on experiences and attitudes of 12 to 15 year olds.* London: HMSO.

Ball, S., Maguire, M., and Macrae, S., 2000. *Choice, pathways and transitions post-16: new youth, new economies in the global city.* London: Routledge/Falmer.

BBC 2003. Gun crime growing like cancer. BBC News, 21 May. Available from: http://news.bbc.co.uk/1/hi/england/3043701.stm [Accessed 8 April 2008].

Beck, U., 1992. *Risk society.* London: Sage.

Becker, H., 1963. *Outsiders: studies in the sociology of deviance.* New York: The Free Press.

Blackman, S., 2005. Youth subcultural theory: a critical engagement with the concept, its origins and politics, from the Chicago school to postmodernism. *Journal of youth studies*, 8 (1), 1–20.

Bose, M., 2003. 'Race' and class in the post-industrial economy. *In*: D. Muggleton and R. Weinzierl, eds. *The post-subcultural reader.* Oxford: Berg, 167–180.

Bowling, B. and Phillips, C., 2002. *Racism, crime and justice.* Harlow: Pearson Education.

Brunson, R. and Miller, J., 2006. Young black men and urban policing in the United States. *British journal of criminology*, 46 (4), 613–640.

Bullock, K. and Tilley, N., 2008. Understanding and tackling gang violence. *Crime prevention and community safety*, 10, 36–47.

Burrell, S., 1990. Gang evidence: issues for criminal defense. *Santa Clara law review*, 30 (3), 739–790.

Cahill, C., 2000. Street literacy: urban teenagers' strategies for negotiating their neighbourhood. *Journal of youth studies*, 3 (3), 251–277.

Calhoun, C., 1991. Indirect relationships and imagined communities: large-scale social integration and the transformation of everyday life. *In*: P. Bourdieu and J.S. Coleman, eds. *Social theory for a changing society.* Boulder, CO: Westview, 95–121.

Chesney-Lind, M., Rockhill, A., Marker, N., and Reyes, H., 1994. Gangs and delinquency. *Crime, law, and social change*, 21 (3), 201–228.

Cloward, R. and Ohlin, L., 1960. *Delinquency and opportunity.* London: Routledge and Kegan Paul.

Cohen, A.K., 1955. *Delinquent boys.* Glencoe, IL: The Free Press.

Cohen, S., 1972. *Moral panics and folk devils.* London: McGibbon and Kee.

Cohen, S., 1979. The punitive city: notes on the dispersal of social control. *Crime, law and social change*, 3 (4), 339–363.

Collins, D. and Kearns, K., 2001. The safe journey of an enterprising school: negotiating landscapes of opportunity and risk. *Health and place*, 7, 293–306.

Downes, D., 1966. *The delinquent solution.* London: Routledge & Kegan Paul.

Esbensen, F., Winfree, L., He, N., and Taylor, T., 2001. Youth gangs and definitional issues: when is a gang a gang, and why does it matter? *Crime and delinquency*, 47 (1), 105–130.

Fagan, J. and Tyler, T.R., 2005. Legal socialization of children and adolescents. *Social justice research*, 18 (3), 217–241.

Flood-Page, C., Campbell, S., Harrington, V., and Miller, J., 2000. *Youth crime: findings from the 1998/99 youth lifestyles survey.* London: Home Office Research, Development and Statistics Directorate.

Fraser, P., 1996. Social and spatial relationships and the 'problem' inner city. *Critical social policy*, 16 (49), 43–65.

Garland, D., 2001. *The culture of control.* Oxford: Oxford University Press.

Giddens, A., 1991. *Modernity and self-identity: self and society in the late modern age.* Cambridge: Polity.

Guardian, 2005. The trials of living with the feral youths of Salford. *Guardian*, 21 May. Available from: http://www.guardian.co.uk/society/2005/may/21/youthjustice.classroomviolence [Accessed 8 April 2008].

Hagedorn, J., 1988. *People and folks: gangs, crime and the underclass in a rust belt city.* Chicago: Lake View Press.

Hagedorn, J., 1990. Back in the field again: gang research in the nineties. *In*: C.R. Huff, ed. *Gangs in America.* Newbury Park, CA: Sage, 240–262.

Hall, T., Coffey, A., and Williamson, H., 1999. Self, space and place: youth identities and citizenship. *British journal of the sociology of education*, 20 (4), 501–513.

Hallsworth, S. and Young, T., 2004. Getting real about gangs. *Criminal justice matters*, 55 (1), 12–13.

Home Office, 2004. *Code of practice for the exercise by police officers of statutory powers of stop and search (Code A).* London: Home Office.

Home Office, 2008. *Tackling gangs: a practical guide for local authorities, CDRPs and other local partners.* London: Home Office.

Katz, C., Webb, V., and Schaefer, D., 2000. The validity of police gang intelligence lists: examining differences in delinquency between documented gang members and nondocumented delinquent youth. *Police quarterly*, 3 (4), 413–437.

Katz, C. and Webb, V., 2006. *Policing gangs in America.* New York: Cambridge University Press.

Kintrea, K., Bannister, J., Pickering, J., Reid, M., and Suzuki, N. 2008. *Young people and territoriality in British cities.* York: Joseph Rowntree Foundation.

Klein, M., 1995. *The American street gang.* New York: Oxford University Press.

Lemert, E., 1951. *Social pathology.* New York: McGraw-Hill.

MacDonald, R., Shildrick, T., Webster, C., and Simpson, D., 2005. Growing up in poor neighbourhoods: the significance of class and place in the extended transitions of 'socially excluded' adults. *Sociology*, 39 (5), 873–891.

Marshall, M., Frazer, S., Smith, I., Fuller, C., Geddes, M., Ardron, R., *et al.*, 2004. *Young people in NDC areas: findings from six case studies.* Research Report 20, New Deal for Communities National Evaluation. Sheffield: Sheffield Hallam University.

McAra, L. and McVie, S., 2005. The usual suspects?: street-life, young people and the police. *Criminal justice*, 5 (1), 5–36.

McConville, M., Sanders, A., and Leng, R., 1991. *The case for the prosecution.* London: Routledge.

McConville, M., Sanders, A., and Leng, R., 1997. Descriptive or critical sociology – the choice is yours. *British journal of criminology*, 37 (4), 347–58.

McCorkle, R. and Miethe, T., 1998. The political and organizational response to gangs: an examination of a 'moral panic' in Nevada. *Justice quarterly*, 15 (1), 41–64.

Miller, W., 1958. Lower class culture as a generating milieu for gang delinquency. *Journal of social issues*, 14, 5–19.

Parachini, A. and Crew, J., 1996. Memoranda to Mr. Erik S. Brown with the US Commission on Civil Rights (unpublished document).

Parker, H., 1974. *View from the boys: a sociology of down-town adolescents.* Newton Abbot: David and Charles Holding.

Pitts, J., 2008. Describing and defining youth gangs. *Community safety journal*, 7 (1), 26–31.
Quinton, P., Bland, N. and Miller, J., 2000. *Police stops, decision-making and practice*. Police Research Series Paper No. 130. London: Home Office.
Reiner, R., 1997. Policing and the police. *In*: M. Maguire, R. Morgan and R. Reiner, eds. *The Oxford handbook of criminology*. 2nd edn. Oxford: Oxford University Press, 997–1050.
Scarman, Lord, 1981. *The Scarman Report: the Brixton disorders*, Cmnd 8427. London: HMSO.
Sharp, D. and Atherton, S., 2007. To serve and protect?: The experiences of policing in the community of young people from black and other ethnic minority groups. *British journal of criminology*, 47 (4), 746–763.
Shaw, C.R. and McKay, H., 1942. *Juvenile delinquency and urban areas*. Chicago: University of Chicago Press.
Shildrick, T. and MacDonald, R., 2006. In defence of subculture: young people, leisure and social divisions. *Journal of youth studies*, 9 (2), 125–140.
Smith, D.J., 1991. Police and racial minorities. *Policing and society*, 2 (1), 1–16.
Spergel, I., 1995. *The youth gang problem*. New York: Oxford University Press.
Sullivan, M., 2005. Maybe we shouldn't study 'gangs': does reification obscure youth violence? *Journal of contemporary criminal justice*, 21 (2), 170–190.
The Sun, 2006. 500,000 hoodies in gangs. 26 May.
Thrasher, F., 1927. *The gang*. Chicago: University of Chicago Press.
Tita, G., Cohen, J., and Engberg, J., 2005. An ecological study of the location of gang 'set space'. *Social problems*, 52 (2), 272–299.
Venkatesh, S.A., 1997. The social organization of street gang activity in an urban ghetto. *American journal of sociology*, 103 (1), 82–111.
Vigil, J.D., 2002. *A rainbow of gangs: street cultures in the mega-city*. Austin, TX: University of Texas Press.
White, R., 1996. No-go in the fortress city: young people, inequality and space. *Urban policy and research*, 14 (1), 37–50.
Young, T., FitzGerald, M., Hallsworth, S., and Joseph, I., 2007. *Groups, gangs and weapons*. London: Youth Justice Board.
Youth Justice Board, 2007. Rod Morgan leaves the Youth Justice Board, 26 January 2007. Available from: http://www.yjb.gov.uk/en-gb/News/RodMorganleavestheYJB.htm [Accessed 6 April 2008].

'Nightscapes and leisure spaces': an ethnographic study of young people's use of free space

Cara Robinson

Young Persons' Drug and Alcohol Service, Canterbury, UK, and Department of Media, Canterbury Christ Church University, Canterbury, UK

Space is a good starting point for ethnographic study into youth, as it sets the stage in which dramas unfold. The paper will argue that space should be considered as a character itself – a member of the group whose actions should form part of data collection. For space acts as initiator: in space other issues can evolve and occur. In space, risk-taking behaviours transpire. Space bears witness to crime and conceals drug use. In it, embodiment is progressed – it endorses transition. It also portrays and signifies the social exclusion and marginalization of youth. This article will highlight that the space and place of the street or park is instrumental in the establishment of youth identity. Nightscapes and leisure spaces form an essential character in youth history, acting as creator of memory and enabling transition from one state to another.

Introduction

This paper is taken from a PhD thesis into substance use, deviancy and social exclusion among young people (Robinson 2009). The study is interdisciplinary, incorporating sociology, social anthropology, cultural studies and criminology. The empirical research is informed by and makes a contribution to the theoretical debate on risk, nightscapes and leisure spaces appropriated by young people; in particular the study advances the ideas of body projects, telling stories and liminality. Illegal drug use by young people is a contentious area that attracts much public, political and academic debate. My thesis makes a deeper exploration into the issue of drug use among youth by situating young people's drug-taking behaviour within the contexts of space and place, the body, gender and risk. The thesis is relevant for it considers young people's accounts of their experiences and their attempts to manage and resolve life transitions.

This paper takes as its focus the issue of nightscapes and leisure spaces in relation to youth. It undertakes a selective reading of the relevant literature in these areas and applies theory to the experiences of the research participants, using ethnography as the method in which to elicit young people's stories. The paper explores how street and park spaces are complex systems offering the chance of transition development to those who offer such spaces their time and commitment. I then consider the polarization of free space and consumerized spaces within the lives of young people and look at free space as an important factor in the creation and organization of familiar local knowledge. Spaces are testing and I will explore issues of ownership of space. I am particularly interested in the duality that can exist in space: the public versus the private. Youth activities within free space have attracted societal fear and concern. Attempts to monitor street-based leisure have seized upon surveillance as a tool to control space and youth, yet this approach to youth fails to acknowledge the importance of free space within transition development (MacDonald and Marsh 2005). Finally, the paper looks at the concept of liminality as a useful tool to explain the condition of youth.

Fieldwork, the 'White House Group' and the observer

Four groups of young people participated in the research, occupying three different geographical locations in the south of England as leisure space. This paper will consider one of these groups: the 'White House Group', who occupied a park space in the centre of a seaside town. The White House Group was the first group that I entered into fieldwork with. My engagement with the group was eased by my practitioner status. During my research I also continued to work as drug and alcohol specialist treatment coordinator for the KCA (UK) Young Persons' Service. My knowledge of the drug and alcohol field meant that I was able to engage the young people in conversation about their illicit activities. However, this did not prepare me for entering the fieldwork setting, away from the comforts of the counselling room.

From my conversations with young people as a drug/alcohol practitioner, I had become aware of the importance of their leisure time within the free spaces of streets and parks. Street and park spaces can be recognized as complex systems in the formulation of youth histories (MacDonald and Marsh 2005). In order to assert history on a space, it must first be identified and claimed by youth. Barriers hinder and limit young people's appropriation of space. The fieldwork led me to consider group activity within free leisure spaces and to compare this with young people's experiences of statutory youth clubs and commercialized spaces. From data collection I found that increasing social division exists within the night-time economy. Despite being unable legally to access adult activities, young people find themselves having to navigate pathways through a landscape of commodified images in order to assert a sense of identity. Street and park spaces have the attraction of being able to generate memory, facilitating information for future reference (Bourdieu 1984, Crouch and Matless 1996). Spaces are testing, however, and interaction in such space comes at a price – often involving a degree of risk. The embodiment of street spaces and the presence of young people utilizing street and park spaces act to alter the substance of space. Young people's use of public space is often contentious. The use of space is often multi-layered with purpose and function, and young people have to manage the shrinking of accessible space within an increasing surveillance society (Crouch 1998). Given such complexities, young people's utilization of free space is complex and often misunderstood.

I studied the young people who formed the White House Group at their local meeting place – a park. The group with whom I engaged from March until September 2004 consisted of four females and eight males, aged 15 and 16 years. For the purposes of confidentiality, the group provided me with already established pseudonyms that they had for one another. The group were known to the early intervention drug and alcohol worker (KCA, UK), who was able to introduce me to individuals. The group had been highlighted by their school as being vulnerable to substance misuse. The group were keen for me to observe them at the White House (local park) and were active in describing and showing me their use of substances. The group welcomed me into their space and were willing to engage with the research – all bar one young female ('Smiley'), who immediately took on the role of gatekeeper. Only 'Smiley' proved to be suspicious of my intentions. The others' acceptance meant that newcomers to the group during the period of observation automatically did not question my position within the group. Relations were quickly formed, and it was not long before members of the group felt that they needed to test the boundaries with me. The young people were keen for me to smoke cannabis with them. When I declined their offers early in our relationship, they would attempt to blow smoke over me so that I might be intoxicated by proxy and therefore party to the illicit act. They also asked me to purchase alcohol for them – this was also refused. Our relationship was appeased by my use of food as a bargaining tool (Blackman 2007, p. 707). I would swap doughnuts and pizza for conversation and data. The group liked this research tool, as it also helped with their cannabis-induced 'munchies' (cannabis has the effect of lowering blood sugar levels, often making the user incredibly hungry). The young people were at times capable of going to some lengths to ensure that I achieved 'good copy' – data that arrived from the young people managing what they felt I wanted to learn. The research location was chosen by my personal preference for 'comfort areas', night-time locations where I felt comfortable. Ethical considerations were also taken into account so that my research areas and practitioner locations did not overlap. My practitioner role has meant that over the last seven years I have gained considerable empathy for the issues facing young substance users. This empathic role has led to an interesting nuance where I can speak with young people about private and deviant behaviour that is not easily revealed to adult society while also being afforded distance from the issue. Much consideration was given to role-conflict issues prior to the fieldwork taking place. The White House Group was made up of young people who resided in two different geographical locations – their commitment to getting to the space often proved ingenious and steadfast, involving the invention of stories to parents in order to gain funds for public transport. This group commitment meant that their associations in the park were not loosely based or transient, but rather that the young people were forming substantial relationships with one another over a period of time. The young people had been meeting in the park on a regular basis for two years. When questioned about their relationships with one another, the young people often spoke of their peers as 'family', and there were times during personal crisis when individuals chose to seek out their peers, rather than seek advice or support from adults. The group were made up of young people from various backgrounds. One of the young males came from an affluent family. Others reported family breakdown where one parent had moved away from the family unit, thus leaving one parent to run the household. Available financial resources varied among the group, and this affected the group's decision to purchase drugs. Often the group would pool their funds.

The White House space

The park runs parallel to the high street in a seaside town. It consists of well-kept flowerbeds and gardens, and a children's play park. Imposing on this space is the

'White House' – a large, council-run building of four storeys. Alongside this is a newer building constructed as a day centre for the elderly. The 'White House' offices are functional and unremarkable during the daytime. At night, the space transforms into an illicit leisure place where a hidden group of young people meet. During my time with the group, no other party bore witness to their activities or invaded the space. I received information early in the process from the local police that they were monitoring activities in the park, but I saw no evidence of this. Throughout the data collection, I was aware that illegal acts (drug taking) often occurred. Cohen and Young (1981) suggest that drug-taking communities strengthen their organization when the police intensify their action within an area. A rise in police action, Cohen and Young claim, heightens the need for drug users to segregate themselves from the wider society of non-drug users. It was clear at an early stage, from observing the group smoking drugs (cannabis) openly in a space that was exposed to outside forces, that either drug use had become normalized among the group, or taking risks had become an important part of being within the space. The group were in the process of becoming aware that their drug-taking behaviour was not such a secret activity – but they nevertheless continued their use of drugs. Being associated with drug taking acted as a symbol of difference and also functioned as a ritualistic process, with those accomplished at rolling a 'joint' (cannabis cigarette) having increased kudos among their fellow peers.

The steps at the front of the White House building act as a congregating place where young people can sit. The alleyways that run around the building would today be considered poorly designed, as they allow space for interactions between young people. In a society where Anti-Social Behaviour Orders mean much media coverage, the White House is a space that could be a site for moral panic. Hiding space, space for private interaction, is afforded by the White House. The park is a distinctive place – it does not have the restricting boundaries of a youth club, and the space is not controlled by statutory agencies with imposing agendas. It is not a space where behaviour is subdued or affected by adult authority. Peer interactions determine what occurs there. Risk is perceived and measured in this space, and ritualism ensures a distinct separation between the impetuousness of youth and the rationality of adulthood. There is an element of positive choice about 'the street' as a venue for action – it is free in commercial terms (although the drugs used to keep the space entertaining come at a price) and free in terms of close control. The space guarantees the possibility of a range of differing actions. Most importantly, young people make the decisions on what they want to do, when they want to do it, and when they want to stop it. It can be argued that 'street time' is the only space in a young person's development and transition from youth to adulthood where the opportunity to test fully autonomy over actions is obtainable. It is a far cry from the institutionalization of the youth club, which speaks of limitations to young people. There is a contradiction between the youth clubs' need to reach young people and the need to change young people's behaviour in some way. The youth club gives an appearance of freedom, which is soon denied. Young people who are 'hidden' make this connection very quickly.

Street spaces can be marked out: the White House Group had defined their space through marking it. A large cartoon character smoking a cannabis bong has been scribed on the wall with the words: 'Jim pulled a bong ere' (Jim's bong was a self-made device, using a plastic bottle, in which to smoke cannabis). Graffiti exist around the alleyways – the group understanding who wrote what and why (Jim was quick to point out to me that, as he was busy 'pulling a bong' at the time, he could not have written it). The graffiti act to draw out the perimeters of the space; they also record the young people's history. It is a complex space in that it breeds a need to strike out on one's own even if this entails a level of deception, yet it also necessitates a degree of respect – the group informed me that they would not entertain smashing the windows of the council offices for amusement. It is an 'in-your-face' space that has drawn police attention. From time to time the police attempt to regulate what occurs there, but there can be no doubt that the space cannot be understood or fully realized by those outside its night-time parameters. No adult had accessed the group before to document the nature of the interactions that occur there. It is the interactions that occur within this space that form part of the ethnography. Activities that occur in parks tend to be self-generated; in this respect, activities are uncultivated by organization and are oblivious of commercial significance. Crouch (1994) and Comedia (1995) consider that this affords people the opportunity to discover a captivating space of possibility. Young people do not frequent the streets as individuals; they do so together, often bringing quite different knowledge with them.

Space is a social product, or a complex social construction, that shapes perceptions and spatial practices, based on values and the social production of meanings (Lefebvre 1991). Lefebvre proposes that geographical space needs to be understood as fundamentally social and he highlights the importance of lived experience. Harvey (1973) argues that 'The question "What is space?" [must] ... be replaced by the question "how is it that distinctive human practices create and make use of distinctive spaces?"' (p. 14). He contends that social practices generate space, and in turn these spaces enable, modify and constrain those practices.

The topography of the street acts as a medium for social encounters. Streets are sites of political protest, of power and resistance. The street is identifiable – within the local landscape, yet it reveals broader cultural and social processes. Social identities and social practices are shaped by street experience. Crouch (1998) questions whether increasing social control will mean the end of the street as 'public space'. In our day-to-day lives, we tend to disregard the familiar iconographies of the street. The street is a place of consumption; it is also a place to gaze and be gazed at: for the surveilling and the surveilled. The street is an area of display and also a place that offers detachment. The young people rejoiced in seeing others in the space, but also found enjoyment in being seen.

Free space versus consumerized space

Chatterton and Hollands (2003) state that increased polarization exists within the night-time economy:

> In the shadows of the bright neon of youthful gentrified nightlife consumption, there exists the 'residue' of near-forgotten groups, community/public spaces and traditional drinking establishments marginalized by new urban brandscapes and the commercial mainstream. (Chatterton and Hollands, 2003, p. 175).

Chatterton and Hollands claim that nightscapes for the affluent and self-indulgence sit uncomfortably alongside less desirable spaces of the street and the park. They state that in such areas excluded young people are clinging 'on to the vestiges of non-commercialised public space' (2003, p. 175), and point to films such as *Trainspotting* (Danny Boyle 1996) as a representation of how youth groups are displaced and disaffected. Chatterton and Hollands argue that both the spaces and the young people themselves are surplus to requirements in a new emerging 'post-industrial corporate landscape, replete with its themed fantasy world of excessive hedonism and forceful consumer power' (2003, p. 175).

The participants' actions in their park suggested that they were indeed clinging on to a space they had worked to claim as their own. The group had located this space outside the wider space of the area's night-time economy and had drawn up systems for when this space should be accessed. Other commercial night-time spaces were available to the young people depending on available funds and resources. An adult nightclub out of town ('The Fridge') held fortnightly under-16 nights to which several of the young people were drawn. Going to the nightclub entailed different rituals from those associated with the park. A different dress code was required, and entrance requirements meant that the young people had to adjust their behaviour. Heavy staffing meant that the club would not allow entry to any young person considered under the influence of substances. This meant having to carefully administer the right amount of substances prior to going into the club, in order to avoid detection. Going to the club also meant that the group would come into contact with other young people from other areas. The girls commented that the boys tended to act 'differently' in the club – they noted that the boys would find a space in the club and stand there, viewing the scene. The girls stated that the boys would not dance. There was a general feeling among the group that the club did not meet their needs. The music targeted young people (playing 'S Club 7' and Peter Andre) but failed to reflect the needs of the group, whose musical tastes tend to reflect 'life on the streets' (such as hip hop and drum and bass).

The group attended 'The Fridge' on several occasions throughout the observation. In discussion the group reflected on their need to access adult consumer night space. It was as if the promise of an adult environment lured them to the club, yet the heavy-handed door staff treatment, the selling only of soft drinks, and the youth-tailored music, along with the silliness of other younger people in the club, failed to deliver the promise of adult excitement. The young persons' nightclub seemingly had the same faults as the statutory youth club. The group were also concerned about 'getting there too soon', meaning that they were concerned about experiencing adult sensations too soon. If they got into the club and pub scene now, it may fail to have any allurement when they reach the magic age of 18. Despite the experience of 'The Fridge', the young people continued to be drawn to the space of the street. Commodification and the images that it bears upon young people cannot be ignored (Chatterton and Hollands 2003, p. 176). 'The Fridge' experience highlights that the young people hold metaphors of commodification within the 'real space' of the park. Young people negotiate a landscape of commodified images and appropriate such images to assert street credibility. The fieldwork noted that the young people manipulated materials to suit their own needs – images of consumption offer young people vehicles for interpreting their world. Commodities (such as drugs/alcohol) become symbols (representing adult life) that add meaning to original experience. Such symbols, while being based in the adult world, contrarily are often inexplicable to adults. Codes and systems are reworked and combined in order to provide original meaning relevant to the experience of that particular group. Images of the commodified landscape bring into play a further element that requires investigation. The fieldwork revealed that young people in a masterly way appropriate commodified images to suit their needs, and these images clearly hold social significance in terms of 'moral panic' – however, it would be foolish to overlook the complex nature of the relationship between the street and young people and relate it entirely their use of commodified symbols. The street moves beyond being merely a space in which to consume (alcohol/drugs) and becomes a catalyst for the creation of memory.

Space as a creator of memory

The young people's actions in the street (or park) can be seen as endeavours to maximize the chances that they will be involved in something extraordinary and significant – events creditable for remark and remembrance. This means that long periods of time are spent seemingly 'hanging around' and 'doing nothing' while, on closer inspection, young people are busy conversing, telling stories and planning future activities (Corrigan 1976). Youth clubs rarely offer this experience free from adult intervention. When the night space fails to deliver the promise of noteworthy events, the place is perpetuated by the chance that next week such an event will occur. This chance lures young people to the space: the possibility of missing a 'historical' event ensures that the young people return to the park. The young people recalled stories of events that had occurred in the space. The summer before the research, some of the young men in the group had engaged in competition of who could consume the most Ecstasy tablets in one session. They also spoke about the evening when they had tried their first cannabis bong. Memories of events in the space were not always pleasant. The group were mindful that their drug-taking behaviour had resulted in some of the young men assaulting two young, foreign exchange students, leading to criminal prosecution. Although it can be interpreted as a dangerous space, the park is also a comfortable one. It is recognizable, consistent and historical. The street is a series of fragmented and broken parts – each part is its own site, telling its own story. The street acts as a familiar organizer of local knowledge (Bourdieu 1984, Crouch and Matless 1996). It is the provider of memories of past interactions – it charts people and contains and triggers memories, anecdotes, hopes and encounters. Places become embodied with systems and knowledge, memories of the street inform the future. In this sense the place takes on its own character and the street becomes significant in ordinary, lived experience. The character of the street takes on an identity of shared interest. Streets are sites where crucial events occur – events cut across, depart from and spill on to streets and become local myth. The character is forever changing in terms of literal environment – but irrespective of the physical challenges it imposes, the young people's interactions with it are adaptable (such as having to adapt according to seasons and weather). Throughout the period of observation, it was noted that the young people displayed much durability and hardiness. Durability and hardiness are necessary among youth in order that they can make claims on their street and their lives. Their resilience often exceeded my own; long periods of fieldwork time were spent in cold, dark, rainy conditions.

Testing places and contending spaces

'The street' has no definite boundary or border – it extends beyond physical buildings and is fluid. Crouch (1998) maintains that to understand images of the street it is necessary to be there at its margins, to see what happens in the corners. Representations of place are made up partly in terms of leisure practices. Leisure aims to serve enjoyment and identity, it fulfils the need for consumption and aids empowerment. Engagement in leisure practices can also involve opposition, resistance and transgression. Parks feed life to 'the street' – the park extends the world of 'the street' and makes its edges ambiguous (Willats 1982, Crouch 1989, 1994, Willis 1990, Nielsen 1995). Activities can spill over from the park and enter 'the street'. The space of the park can be measured from 'the street': actions that occur in the park influence the meaning of the street to those who use the park or choose to pass by. It can be a welcoming or a dangerous place and is often synonymous with youth moral panic. Willis (1990) conducted a study of young people on the streets and found that the street acted as a conveyor of their activities. The street not only functioned as a physical meeting place but also embodied meanings and metaphors relevant to the young people's lives. It was a container of escape and diversion but also represented home. The street yielded opportunity – a place to be seen and to view others. In this respect the street becomes a place of sharing, a confrontational challenging space, but one that promises ownership for those who put the time and effort into claiming it – especially after dark.

Ownership of the 'Whitehouse' space appeared multi-layered, and there seemed to be a sense of duality surrounding the space: public versus private space. It was council owned during the day, and there was attempted governance by police at night alongside the young people's appropriation of the space. Even among the group studied, there were other contenders: young people were observed on the periphery of the dominant group – attempting assimilation and lying in wait to stake their claim on the space. During one evening, a group of girls stood in the park close to the group. They gradually edged closer and closer until the group, rather uninterested in the younger girls, decided to move on from the space. Interestingly, they asked me to accompany them – stressing a need to escape the young girls' advances. The 'White House Group' afterwards reflected that once they had moved on from the space, outgrown its capacities for excitement and fun, a new generation would be ready to take their place. In this respect the space becomes self-perpetuating – ensuring development of its history. It appeared that there were always new stories to be made, but only those of true significance proved lasting. An example of this was the young people's story of the night that they graffitied the wall with a picture of a bong. The young people recounted their group experience of 'pulling a bong' in the space and becoming stoned. It was remembered as a good night as several of the boys got stoned, while the girls consumed alcohol. Barney remembered it as the first time that she had tried a bong and then had 'got off with Jim'. Barney recounted events of this evening as pivotal in her forming a lasting relationship with Jim. Graffiti served to provide a marker of an event to be remembered and identified the place as belonging to the group. As one young person, Biscuit, pointed out, it 'sets the trademark – we've been there.'

Other characters operated within the space – and were allowed to move freely to share the park. The group often spoke of an intravenous heroin user who shared the park space in order to 'jack-up'. Derogatory terms were used to describe this adult, and he functioned as a constant indicator of problematic drug use. Such drug use was described as being poles apart from the young people's drug use. However, one member of the group was pessimistic about the group's future: 'Droop' stated that he felt that several members of the group would inevitably end up using heroin. He judged that he would be one of the people most likely to try heroin. The young people were keen to experiment with new drugs; however, heroin was a drug outside the young people's self-boundaries that existed. 'Droop', when questioned about his prediction, concluded that he felt it would be an inevitable consequence of the group's keenness to experiment with drugs.

MacDonald and Marsh (2005) highlight the fact that relatively few studies consider criminal and drug-use careers alongside an exploration of youth leisure to chronicle youth transitions. They were surprised when gathering their data about the significance of incorporating young people's accounts of their leisure time in their study. They found that young people's leisure pursuits enabled a better understanding of their current life situations. The large majority of their research participants spent most of their leisure time 'hanging around' in public spaces. Attempts to monitor street-based youth cultures have been hostile (Anti-Social Behaviour Orders, curfews) and have overshadowed the importance that street-based leisure and unsupervised time has on the formation of youth identity.

Historically, groups of young people gathering on street corners have been commonly regarded as being disorderly and deviant – and therefore should be monitored, protested about, and dispersed by adult authority (Pearson 1983). The group of young people observed, rejected this viewpoint and argued that, apart from their substance use, their behaviour was not deviant but symptomatic of youth. In interview, Chelsea informed me that she believed that adults in the town where she lives see her as 'troublesome':

CR: How do you think other people see you?
Chelsea: Adults see me as troublesome. Since a happy slapping incident was on the local news it's affected how others view us hanging around in a group. The other day an old lady saw us walking along the street and crossed over the road. People are always walking round us.

The White House Group were keen to tell me that their group was made up of a mixture of personalities – some young people whose behaviour had led them to be permanently excluded from school, some whose behaviour had put them on restricted programmes in an attempt to keep them in school, some who were known to the local youth-offending service, and some who were doing well at school. Each young person had a clearly stated role within the group. Giggles was known as the 'straight member of the group' – choosing to abstain from drugs and alcohol – and was relied upon to recall noteworthy events. Giggles was looked upon to 'sort out' the others while drunk or stoned. Barney's role was to take care of Jim and ensure that he did not 'lose it' (lose his temper, become paranoid), Sparrow and Droop were the entertainers in terms of how much drugs they could consume in one evening, and Josh was replied upon to pool the funds and to liaise with their drug dealer. The young people saw the involvement of all members of the group as essential to its status and purpose, each young person having a part to play in the development of its history.

Across the fieldwork, it became clear that individuals retained a sense of belonging to their chosen space. Loader (1996) argues that young people's continual use of familiar public space and the development of localized identity can be seen as a wider indication of marginalized transitions. In his study of youth in Edinburgh, Loader writes:

> Denied the purchasing power needed to use, or even to get to, other parts of the city (and most importantly the city centre) unemployed youths are for the most part confined to the communities in which they live ... as a result, the 'locality' tends to retain a prominent place in the lives of marginalized young people, both as a site of routine activities and as the basis of their identities .... Hanging around the streets becomes a culturally inappropriate way of killing endless time. (Loader 1996, pp. 112–113)

Attempts to control space

Chatterton and Hollands (2003, p. 70) note societal attempts to clean up and regulate public space, describing 'a general sanitisation of activity through increased surveillance'.

There have been extensive accounts of concern surrounding troublesome street youth in the UK (Corrigan 1976, Pearson 1983, Muncie 1999). More recently, there have been a number of 'moral panics' regarding young people's disruptive use of public space – in parks, on estates, playing fields and street corners (Jeffs and Smith 1996, Loader 1996, Stenson and Watts 1998, MacDonald and Marsh 2002). In 2000, 2000a survey of communities argued that 'On all estates, and across all age groups, the biggest single issue identified by respondents was the anti-social behaviour of children and teenagers' (Page 2000, p. 37).

How, then has society sought to manage fear of anti-social behaviour among communities? Throughout the period of observation, the layout of public parks has been of considerable interest. In many parks, alongside children's playgrounds there are 'youth shelters'. These are metal constructions consisting of a roof to protect against adverse weather conditions, and seating. They exist as a place for young people to congregate. A website for 'People United Against Crime' a registered charity founded by South Yorkshire Police, campaigns for proactive measures to counteract anti-social behaviour. They boast that

> People United Against Crime's contribution to combating anti-social behaviour is to work with local communities throughout South Yorkshire to provide more facilities for young people. Through the provision of amenities such as youth shelters, multi-use games areas, skate parks and an Internet Café, we have been able to engage young people and move them to recreational areas where they are less intimidating to the wider community.

The aim to move young people to specified areas is of concern to me – the youth shelters studied during fieldwork were often in isolated, unlit spaces within parks. It may be that the need to calm moral panic within society is at a cost to the safety and welfare of the young people who use such shelters. The White House Group acknowledged that there were times when the group became separated while intoxicated. Several of the girls informed me that they had on occasion walked home on their own. While drunk the girls did not assess the risks involved. However, in conversation with me and with hindsight, they agreed that this was a risky practice.

Transitions

In the fieldwork the young people's relationship with the street provided a consistent sense of attachment and belonging at a time when transitions were being entered into – for example, in personal relationships and in the home environment. During fieldwork, Nadine was an important member of the White House Group. She was a consistent presence in the park, always drawing attention to herself with her loud and vibrant interactions with her friend Jo, with whom she had a close relationship. Near the end of the period of fieldwork, Nadine fell pregnant following a one-night stand with Goldie, a well-respected member of the group. It was at this time that I was also pregnant. There evolved a contradiction whereby both Nadine and I recognized a similarity of experience and unstoppable move towards a new transition – we were entering the same period of transition in that we were experiencing the same bodily changes, yet there was also an unvoiced appreciation of the differences of our experiences. This was further compounded by the fact that news of Nadine's pregnancy split the group for a period of time. Nadine eventually disengaged from the group and the park. At our last contact, Nadine acknowledged that her life was going to change and her move into adulthood had been unexpectedly advanced. For Nadine, being pregnant meant that she could no longer hang around on the street and in the park. There was an awareness that she could no longer drink large amounts of alcohol and indulge in risk behaviour and she began to acknowledge that her new role as a mother would take her back into the home environment:

> **CR**: How have things been going? Have you been to the White House much?
> **Nadine**: Nah, don't get the chance these days. I've been staying in with my mum talking about baby stuff. Apart from Jo, I don't talk to the group much. Goldie winds me up and I don't want to get into more fights with him case I hurt the baby.

MacDonald and Marsh (2005) in their study of young people in Teesside found that processes of disengagement from street-based leisure often coincided for young women with transitions such as moving into independent housing and/or becoming pregnant.

Liminality

My data collection and thoughts on youth transitions led me to consider liminality as a concept to help describe the condition of youth. Van Gennep (1960) and Turner (1967) in their theories of ritualistic practices describe liminality as the second stage of three stages whereby in a ritual (particularly in a rite of passage) participants experience change – especially change in regard to social status. The liminal state is where a person's sense of identity dissolves to some degree, resulting in disorientation. In fact, the liminal state is characterized by ambiguity, indeterminacy and openness. It is a stage of transition where a person's normal limits to his thoughts, behaviour and understanding of self are relaxed, allowing the possibility of new perspectives to be taken on board. 'Liminal entities are neither here nor there; they are betwixt and between the positions assigned and arrayed by law, custom, convention, and ceremonial' (Turner 1969, p. 95). Liminality can become a permanent state if a transition is not completed. For youth subcultures, interacting factors can produce an enhanced state of liminality. The nature of youth means that young people find themselves in a liminal place between youth and adulthood – struggling to find a clear pathway towards adulthood. Also, the use of narcotic substances induces a liminal state whereby the user becomes located in a place between conscious rationality and unconscious irrationality. Young people often find themselves on the streets and in parks at twilight. Activities cannot take place until after school, and most young people have a time boundary whereby they are expected home at a certain time in the evening – therefore they are unable to stay out all night. Twilight then can be seen as liminal: between day and night. As discussed already, there exists a duality to space and place: places become liminal at night as public space is contested as private space. The White House Group acknowledged police and public disproval of their activities within their chosen sites. In liminal states the familiar becomes unfamiliar, the safe moves towards becoming unsafe. No man's lands and disputed territories become liminal. The 'betweenness' of these spaces defines liminality. For me, the streets and parks that form the source of my data are places to pass through – this aspect of the nature of place was recognizable to the young people observed – they either regretted that when they moved on, others were not visible to take their place or begrudged younger people emerging to stake their claim on the space.

Turner (1967) created the term 'liminoid' to describe experiences liminal in nature – but that are optional and do not entail a resolution of personal crisis. The liminal is a feature of society, while liminoid is a break from society – involving play. Turner argues that liminality is extinct in industrial societies – having been replaced by liminoid experience. We can make a case for liminality within street spaces as society has edged out alternative leisure spaces for young people – who are denied access due to age restrictions or are unable to afford the consumerism that surrounds adult nightscapes. The young people observed and interviewed did not access the nightscapes that had been purposefully designed for them: statutory youth clubs. They had experimented with the activities offered by statutory youth services, but were more likely to be found outside the clubs than inside them. Several of the young people interviewed had been excluded from youth clubs. When the White House Group did attend a youth club (for football practice), their actions in the environment acted to challenge established boundaries. Bam and Gee Gee took great delight in showing me video footage taken on their mobile phones of the group appearing to snort cocaine off the youth club toilet, seemingly representing perceived adult behaviour in pubs/clubs.

The young people on the streets are in a period of transition – struggling to find, enter and resolve a rite of passage to adulthood. The data collection found young people to be experimenting with features of adult life – such as alcohol, money, illicit substances, motor vehicles and sexual relations. While their actions in space may be seen as play and often a violation of societal norms, it is a place that offers identity formation. I wish therefore to propose that young people's appropriation of public spaces is both liminal and liminoid in nature.

Conclusion

My time spent in the field with the White House Group showed me that young people interact with space reflexively. Space has to be contended and ownership negotiated, with young people having to interpret the space and their actions within it.

Storytelling is fundamental to the interpretation of a reflexive project of self – as young people modify existing narratives and form new ones, they undergo transition towards who it is possible to be. Contemporary culture insists that young people actively work towards building self-identity. Throughout the stage of youth, the demand to consider the 'reflexive project of self' (Giddens 1991) materializes in either voluntary form or as a compulsory demand, involving varying degrees of personal control. Storytelling has become a fundamental process of youth. Young people modify existing narratives and form new ones as they undergo transition resolution (McLeod and Thomson 2009). The construction of self is partly generated through public institutions but, more importantly for this paper, it is worked on in private.

The White House park provided the young people with a degree of private space in which to rehearse those adult behaviours perceived by the group as offering facilitation to the changes that each young person was endeavouring to reach. The group were attempting to make the transition from youth to adulthood. Street and park spaces function as space in which to try out and practise new states of self-identity. Such spaces also allow storytelling among peers. For the young person, the street or park allows space within space – space to test out identity, to formulate and assert new self-narratives (Blackman 2007). The street/park therefore is a site of agency and empowerment, which comes at a cost in that by allowing risk, it is also risky. Young people frequenting such nightscapes need to be resilient and hardy. The street and the park are available spaces, allowing young people to come together, despite the ensuing invention of moral panic and folk devils. The dominance of consumerized nightscapes with the need for heavy surveillance has edged out space for young people. Theorists (Blackman 1997, Toon 2000, MacDonald and Marsh 2002) contend that such marginalized space is utilized by underprivileged groups; therefore, increased street surveillance and policing can be seen as a clear assault on youth. My analysis has found that rather than run from or succumb to supervision within their leisure space, young people have found ways to manage and adapt free space in order that it may be used to advance the development of the private self. This has involved interaction within space and reflexivity towards it. How much it is a conscious decision on the part of young people to create and perpetuate space so that it may assist the advancement of self-identity remains unknown; however, what is certain, is that young people will go to great lengths to ensure that their little piece of history is marked on the street.

References

Bauman, Z. and Tester, K., 2001. *Conversations with Zygmunt Bauman*. Cambridge: Polity Press.

Beck, U., 1992. *Risk society: towards a new modernity*. London: Sage.

Blackman, S., 1997. Deconstructing a giro: a critical and ethnographic study of the youth 'underclass'. *In*: R. MacDonald, ed. *Youth, the 'underclass' and social exclusion*. London: Routledge, 113–129.

Blackman, S.J., 2007. Hidden ethnography': crossing emotional borders in qualitative accounts of young people's lives. *Journal of sociology*, 41 (4), 699–716.

Bourdieu, P., 1984. *Distinction: a social critique of the judgement of taste*. London: Routledge.

Chatterton, P. and Hollands, R., 2003. *Urban nightscapes – youth cultures, pleasure spaces and corporate power*. London and New York: Routledge.

Cohen, S. and Young, J., 1981. *The manufacture of news, social problems, deviance and the mass media*. London: Constable.

Comedia, 1995. *Park life.* London and Stroud: Demos-Comedia.
Corrigan, P., 1976. Doing nothing. *In*: S. Hall and T. Jefferson, eds. *Resistance through rituals: youth subcultures in post-war Britain.* London: Hutchinson, 103–105.
Crouch, D., 1994. *The popular culture of city parks.* London and Stroud: Demos-Comedia.
Crouch, D., 1989. Patterns of co-operation in outdoor leisure. *Leisure studies*, 8 (3), 189–199.
Crouch, D., 1998. The street in the making of popular geographical knowledge. *In*: N.R. Fyfe, ed. *Images of the street.* London and New York: Routledge, 160–175.
Crouch, D. and Matless, D., 1996. Refiguring geography: the parish maps of common ground. *Transactions of the Institute of British Geographers*, 21 (1), 236–255.
Giddens, A., 1991. *Modernity and self-identity: self and society in the late modern age.* Cambridge: Polity Press.
Harvey, D., 1973. *Social justice and the city.* London: Arnold.
Henderson, S., Holland, J., McGrellis, S., Sharpe, S., and Thomson, R., 2007. *Inventing adulthoods: a biographical approach to youth transitions.* London: Sage.
Hobbs, D. and May, T., 1993. *Interpreting the field: accounts of ethnography.* Oxford: Clarendon Press.
Jeffs, T. and Smith, M., 1996. Getting the dirtbags off the street: curfews and other solutions to juvenile crime. *Youth and policy*, 53, 1–14.
Lefebvre, H., 1991. *The production of space*, N. Donaldson-Smith, trans. Oxford: Basil Blackwell (original edition 1947).
Loader, I., 1996. *Youth, policing and democracy.* London: Macmillan.
MacDonald, R. and Marsh, J., 2002. Crossing the Rubicon: youth transitions, poverty, drugs and social exclusion. *International journal of drug policy*, 13, 27–38.
MacDonald, R. and Marsh, J., 2005. *Disconnected youth?: growing up in Britain's poor neighbourhoods.* Basingstoke: Palgrave Macmillan.
McLeod, J. and Thomson, R., 2009. *Researching social change: qualitative approaches.* London: Sage.
Muncie, J., 1999. *Youth and crime.* London: Sage.
Nielsen, N.K., 1995. *The stadium and the city: a modern story. In*: J. Bale, ed. *The stadium and the city.* Keele: Keele University Press, 21–44.
Page, D., 2000. *Communities in the balance.* York: Joseph Rowntree Foundation.
Parker, H., Aldridge, J., and Measham, F., 1998. *Illegal leisure: the normalisation of adolescent recreational drug use.* London: Routledge.
Pearson, G., 1983. *Hooligan: a history of respectable fears.* Basingstoke: Macmillan.
Stenson, K. and Watts, P., 1998. The street: 'it's a bit dodgy around there': safety, danger, ethnicity and young people's use of public space. *In*: T. Skelton and G. Valentine, eds. *Cool places: geographies of youth cultures.* London: Routledge.
Toon, I., 2000. 'Finding a place in the street': CCTV surveillance and young people's use of urban public space. *In*: D. Bell and A. Haddour, eds. *City visions.* Harlow: Pearson Education, 141–157.
Turner, V., 1967. Betwixt and between: the liminal period in *rites de passage. In*: *Forest of symbols.* Ithaca, NY: Cornell University Press, 93–111.
Turner, V., 1969. *The ritual process: structure and anti-structure.* Chicago: Aldine.
Van Gennep, A. , 1960. *The rites of passage*, M.B. Vizedom and G.L. Coffee, trans. Chicago: University of Chicago Press.
Whyte, W., 1943. /*1955. Street corner society.* Chicago: University of Chicago Press.
Willatts, S., 1982. *The new reality.* Derry: The Orchard Gallery.
Willis, P., 1990. *Common culture.* Milton Keynes: Open University Press.

Filmography

Trainspotting, 1996. Directed by Danny Boyle.

Grafting, going to college and working on road: youth transitions and cultures in an East London neighbourhood

Anthony Gunter[a] and Paul Watt[b]

[a]*School of Law, University of East London, London, UK;* [b]*Department of Geography, Environment and Development Studies, Birkbeck, University of London, London, UK*

The local neighbourhood has an enduring significance for British urban, working-class youth in relation to their transitions, cultures and leisure practices. This paper examines these interrelated issues by drawing upon ethnographic research undertaken in 'Manor', a deprived, multi-ethnic East London neighbourhood. It explores the transitions taken by black, white and mixed-parentage young males (and some of their female peers), transitions that were formed by the interaction of paid work opportunities with youth cultures and leisure practices ('road' and 'grafter' cultures), ethnicity, gender and social networks. Even within a single deprived and stigmatized neighbourhood such as Manor, a number of transitions could be identified. These include 'grafting' at manual, masculine 'dirty work' in the construction industry; going to college allied to 'clean', service-sector work; and an 'alternative' route of 'working on road' by undertaking a variety of low-level, illegal money-making activities.

Introduction

This paper is concerned with understanding how youth cultures intersect with the transitions and post-16 experiences, choices and opportunities (or lack of) available to black, white and mixed-parentage young males living in a deprived East London neighbourhood. Despite over-arching postmodernist and globalization claims regarding the redundancy of residential space for youth identity formation, the local neighbourhood, including the public space of 'the street', continues to matter for at least *some* groups of young people (Watt and Stenson 1998, MacDonald and Shildrick 2007), notably those from working-class backgrounds growing up in the marginal spaces of Britain's post-industrial cities (see, *inter alia*, Nayak 2003, McDowell 2004). The key research question underpinning this paper is how young males 'from the same locale and from [apparently] the same socio-economic background' (MacDonald *et al.* 2001, p. 5), but different ethnicities, experience the school-to-work transition in relation to their locally generated subculture(s).

Youth transitions and cultures in spaces of urban marginality

Debates over the relative merits of the 'transitions' versus 'cultural' approaches are well rehearsed in the youth studies literature (see, *inter alia*, Cohen and Ainley 2000,

MacDonald *et al.* 2001). This paper acknowledges the criticisms that have been levelled at the youth-as-transitions approach, notably that of being a narrowly economistic interpretation of young people's lives. A preoccupation with the availability (or lack) of waged labour for working-class (especially white male) youth 'led to a limited research paradigm' (Cohen and Ainley 2000, p. 80) that failed to take into account young people's subcultures, identities and leisure activities. However, by offering an account of transitions that takes cultural practices and identities seriously, this paper does not gloss over those structural inequalities that Shildrick and MacDonald (2007) accuse post-subcultural youth studies of neglecting.

The most intensive example of youth transitions research in the UK is that body of work emanating from the University of Teesside (the 'Teesside school'), which has monitored the 'opportunities' for working-class youth living in the marginal neighbourhoods of deindustrialized north-east England (see, *inter alia*, Johnston *et al.* 2000, MacDonald *et al.* 2001, 2005). In broadening the concept of transitions to include 'other' careers apart from school-to-work – for example, criminal careers – the Teesside school has not lost sight of the structural disadvantages facing working-class youth. Notwithstanding its insights, the Teesside school's body of work is nevertheless circumscribed by focusing on white youth in a predominantly 'white place', north-east England (but see Nayak 2003). This begs the question as to how far its approach and findings are relevant to multi-ethnic cities and towns in the UK.

There is considerable evidence that black, Asian and minority ethnic [BAME] young people are subject to persistent labour market disadvantages, partly resulting from exclusionary racist processes, despite higher staying-on rates in schools (Cregan 2002, Bradley 2005). Much of the emphasis within youth labour market research has been placed upon high levels of urban BAME unemployment, as in Liverpool in north-west England (Roberts 1995, pp. 98–99) and London (Fieldhouse 1998). While unemployment is undoubtedly a major problem for BAME youth, it is also important to acknowledge the changing nature and quality of low-level service jobs in the 'new economy', characterized by flexibilization, casualization, informalization and low pay (McDowell 2004, Bradley 2005, Smith, 2005). In her research on how young people experience this new economy in Bristol, south-west England, Bradley (2005) highlights greater BAME youth labour market insecurity and low pay. However, her survey-based research is quite speculative regarding BAME involvement in the variegated interstices of the contemporary urban labour market, notably in relation to 'concealed unemployment' and 'working in the hidden economy' (2005, p. 107). Such gaps highlight the more general limitations of survey data and official statistics in attempting to capture the irregular dynamics of contemporary urban labour markets. This is especially pertinent in relation to what Wacquant (2008, p. 246) refers to as the 'precariat', living in the stigmatized zones of 'advanced marginality' in US and European cities.

In the UK, socio-spatial marginality is often, although not exclusively, identified with deprived inner-city and peripheral social housing estates (Watt 2003, McDowell 2004, Smith 2005). The Teesside school's 'snakes-and-ladders' analysis of the Willowdene council estate in Teesside offers many insights into how young people negotiate their way around locally embedded opportunity structures comprising formal, informal and illegal money-making activities (Johnston *et al.* 2000, MacDonald *et al.* 2001). Two of their conclusions are especially germane to our own analysis here. Firstly, the significance of the locality in shaping youth transitions, and, secondly, the importance of culture whereby no one single youth cultural form operates even in deprived neighbourhoods.

In relation to the neighbourhood, Shildrick and MacDonald (2007) have pointed to the long-standing if unjustly neglected significance of 'street-corner society', which 'remains a central element of working-class *subcultural* identity' for at least some young people (*ibid.*, p. 132; original emphasis). While 'street-corner society' may sound anachronistic, Shildrick and MacDonald's argument is supported by research on the relevance of local public space to youth leisure activities in south-east England, especially for young people from urban black, Asian and white working-class backgrounds (Watt and Stenson 1998). Such a focus on 'the street' is highly relevant to the research findings on 'road culture' in Manor, a deprived multi-ethnic East London neighbourhood, that we report below.

Economic restructuring and 'getting by' in East London

London as a whole has witnessed a profound transformation in its employment profile in the previous 40 years as a result of deindustrialization, decentralization and feminization (Buck *et al.* 2002). Such changes have if anything been even more dramatic in East London, where the development of a post-industrial economy has occurred via the rapid makeover of Docklands into a major financial services hub including extensive gentrification (Hamnett 2003).

Until this relatively recent economic restructuring, East London could be credibly described as a 'one-class city' (Hobbs 1988, p. 86); that is, one dominated by a largely white, manual working class. Historically, the docks and local industries provided physically demanding employment of the masculine 'hard graft' variety, albeit often casualized, while the area's proximity to the Thames meant that enterprising East Enders could by-pass the vagaries of the formal labour market and create their own money-making opportunities (Hobbs 1988). While Hobbs' claim that '*everyone* was "at it"' (1988, p. 8; our emphasis) might be an exaggeration, an informal/illegal economy based upon pilfering and selling stolen goods was well-established by the 1950s in London's East End (Hood and Joyce 1999). By the 1970s–1980s, 'petty crime was regarded as a routine means of raising funds by selling stolen goods in a ready market for "knock off"' (*ibid.*, p. 155), while theft and drug-dealing also became more significant features of working-class life in East London. 'Getting by' through making money via a *variety* of means thus has a long-standing pedigree in East London (Hobbs 1988) and, as we discuss below, remains relevant for contemporary East Londoners.

The transformation of the East London skyline at Canary Wharf and elsewhere in Docklands has not been matched by a similar sea change in the fortunes of its poorer residents, such as those who live in Manor. East London remains one of the poorest regions in the UK and is also increasingly multi-ethnic (Buck *et al.* 2002, Hamnett 2003, LDA 2006). An analysis of the five East London 2012 Olympic host boroughs indicates that worklessness is worse there than in the rest of London and nationally (LDA 2006). Despite aggregate employment growth in East London from the mid-1990s (PACEC 2003, Syrett and North 2008, pp. 69 and 98), there are doubts as to how many of the new jobs, and especially professional-managerial jobs, have gone to locals: 'in London's primary financial centre, Canary Wharf, there are still relatively few people from the locality in employment within the largest concentration of financial services firms in Europe – 15 years after the first firms moved there' (LDA 2006, p. 10). Low-level and no qualifications underpin much of the labour market exclusion and disadvantage in East London (Syrett and North 2008), factors that are worse for young people living there than in the rest of London (LDA 2006). Young people in East London are, for example, more likely to be 'not in employment, education or training' (NEET) than elsewhere in the city (Research as Evidence 2007).

Worklessness, including unemployment and economic inactivity, linked to 'deproletarianization' (Wacquant 2008, p. 26), is undoubtedly a major problem facing deprived groups in East London and London generally, prominent among which are BAME youth (Buck *et al.* 2002). It is not, however, the *only* problem since many of the capital's new post-industrial service jobs as well as older manual jobs are characterized by insecurity, short-termism and low pay due to increased subcontracting and informalization (Abrams 2002, Watt 2003, Smith 2005). A detailed analysis of new jobs in the East London borough of Newham found that the majority were part-time (Syrett and North 2008, pp. 98 and 107), and many East Londoners are employed in low-paid, low-skilled jobs (LDA 2006).

Economic restructuring alongside welfare state neoliberalization has brought increased socio-spatial polarization in London involving gentrification and the enforced concentration of a deprived, multi-ethnic working class into marginal spaces (Watt 2003, 2006, Smith 2005), such as Manor in East London. Hamnett (2003) argues that London's poorest neighbourhoods, dominated by concentrations of social rental housing, represent haunts of an 'outsider surplus population': 'the council [housing] sector is now dominated by those who are not in the labour force, by virtue of either long-term unemployment, retirement, ill-health, disability or single parenthood' (2003, p. 149). While worklessness is a feature of social housing areas in London, including East London (Buck *et al.* 2002), Hamnett fails to capture the interstitial nature and fast-moving dynamics of the city's lower-level labour market by basing his analysis on decennial census statistics. Qualitative research in North London (Watt 2003) and South London (Smith 2005) has unearthed how many residents of council-built estates *do* work in the city's 'flexible' labour market, but that such work often involves shifting combinations of insecure, low-paid, formal and informal employment plus periods of benefit claiming. Thus, unlike Hamnett's one-dimensional notion of a uniformly workless 'outsider surplus population', no work *and* poor work of various forms are intertwined in London's social housing estates, including those that make up Manor. For young men and women growing up in Manor, such opportunities for getting by interact with locally based networks and cultures in fashioning their transitions.

Research in Manor[1]

This paper draws on research data derived from a larger ethnographic youth study (Gunter 2009) undertaken in Manor – a deprived, multi-ethnic East London neighbourhood. Physically, Manor is made up of council and housing association housing stock located in high-rise, tower-block 'sink estates' and a larger number of low-rise estates comprising maisonettes, three-storey apartment blocks and terraced houses. According to the 2001 Census, almost one-third of Manor's residents are in the 'black' Census categories (black Caribbean, black African and black Other). Moreover, more than 40% of Manor's child/youth population is from the black community. As well as being ethnically diverse, Manor is ranked as one of the most deprived neighbourhoods in England (ODPM 2004). Like many East London neighbourhoods, Manor has been the subject of several regeneration schemes, but it remains deprived as well as an area that suffers from considerable stigmatization. However, there is little immediate class polarization since the area around Manor is not, at least not yet, gentrified. Nor is there the same level of white, working-class racism that has beset other East London neighbourhoods (Cohen 1996).

The ethnographic research spanned a 12-month period, although the field researcher (AG) was familiar with many of the young people and the research site, as he had worked in Manor as a detached youth worker for four years prior to the study. The study was undertaken in order to examine the role and significance of contemporary youth subcultures in relation to the transitions and everyday life experiences of particularly, but not exclusively, black young men growing up in one East London neighbourhood. Consequently, just under half of the 53 informants featured in the study were black males, with the remainder of the research sample comprising their black female and white and mixed-parentage (black and white) male and female peers. Semi-structured tape-recorded interviews were undertaken with 22 of the young people, 14 males and eight females, whose ages ranged from 13 to 21. The authors make no claims that the interviewees or the wider study informants are statistically representative of young people either in Manor or in East London generally.[2] Instead, the aim of the paper is to offer a contextualized account of the young people's transitions that locates them firmly within a specific place. In this particular paper, we focus on the transitions made by the black, white and mixed-parentage young males, although reference is also made to their female peers.

Many of the young people (as well as their parents) had been born and brought up in Manor – or near to it – and had built up extensive local kinship and friendship networks. This was not only important for engendering strong local place identities, but also helped with regard to feelings of neighbourhood safety and belonging, findings that resonate with other UK studies of social housing areas (McDowell 2004, MacDonald *et al.* 2005, Watt 2006). The young people lived in a wide variety of household types, but only a small proportion were in a 'traditional' nuclear family. While a few young people lived on their own, most resided with one or other of their parents, usually their mother, along with their siblings.

The majority of the young people's mothers were in either full-time or part-time paid employment outside the home. Their occupations included a mixture of typically female, low-paid routine jobs such as cleaners, shop assistants and dinner ladies, but also low-grade white-collar positions in nursing, social work and local government. A few mothers (all lone parents with younger, dependent children) were registered as unemployed, but worked within the informal 'cash-in-hand' economy as cleaners, carers, dressmakers and waitresses (see also Watt 2003, Smith 2005). Like other deprived London neighbourhoods, Manor was therefore not a 'jobless ghetto' of the type associated with the US inner city (Buck *et al.* 2002, Wacquant 2008), a point that is not irrelevant to how young people negotiate their transitions.

Youth cultures and post-16 transitions in Manor: an overview

Within Manor, 'road culture' is a black-influenced youth subculture that is largely played out in public settings 'on road' [streets] or within those open spaces around the various local housing estates (MacDonald and Shildrick 2007). Road culture in Manor – as is the case with wider black and mainstream British youth cultures – draws heavily upon expressive Black Atlantic popular cultures (Gilroy 1993) that inform the young people's speech styles, dress codes and musical preferences. The authors hesitate to portray road culture in exclusively racial/ethnic terms, as this 'black' reading fails to recognize the participation of large numbers of white and other minority ethnic working-class youth (see also Nayak 2003). Road culture is central to the lives of all the young people growing up in Manor and cuts across ethnicity and gender and – notwithstanding its expressive/aesthetic elements – is largely concerned with the mundaneity of, and attachment to, neighbourhood life. The mundane, everyday nature of the young people's lives in Manor centres on their leisure activities, such as 'catching joke'[3] with their friends or looking to make 'links'[4], playing football or basketball, or 'kotching'[5], or 'passing through'[6] the youth centre.

Grafter youth culture is distinct from road culture since it draws on white, working-class, East London, masculinist traditions, and its adherents are distinguished by their valorization of 'dirty' manual labour ('hard graft') and leisure activities centred on 'going down the pub'. The latter takes over from the 'road' and youth centre as the leisure focal point for the grafters. Grafter culture takes over from road culture in the lives of some young males (mainly white) when they leave school aged 16 and obtain jobs in the construction industry. The female peers of the grafters – in this study, a small group of four young white females who also lived on the Michaels' Estate – were, however, excluded from the key 'work element' of grafter culture as a result of long-term, gendered exclusionary processes operating within construction in London.[7] On leaving school at age 16, these young women also entered the labour market, but they obtained low-paid, non-skilled employment as machine operators in local, small-scale clothes and food-processing factories. However, within a year, three of the young women became pregnant and gave up their jobs to look after their babies. The young women's leisure activities also shifted away from 'on road' towards nightclubs and pubs.

While road culture and grafter cultures are distinct during the post-16 transitions phase, they are not hermetically sealed off from, or antagonistic to, each other, as movement between the two is both fluid and commonplace due to inter-ethnic friendships and alliances (see also Watt and Stenson 1998).

> **dj Wildstyle** [black male, aged 21]: Even now with like my white friends, even though they're in with us [road culture] they've still got that different thing going on, like you go to work… go to the pub straight after work in your work clothes. It's never like an office job.
> **David** [black male, aged 21]: It's like, I'm going graftin', ennit?
> **dj Wildstyle**: That is the term, grafters, they're grafters…. Hence we do electrical installation, we paint and decorate, we do roofing … get up at six in the morning … in the pub all weekend, eat the Sunday roast.

However, in Manor, most of the respondents' closest friends tended to match their own ethnic background, as found by Reynolds (2007) in her study of young, black, British, Caribbean people's friendship networks.

The overwhelming majority of young informants in Manor left school at age 16 with few or no formal qualifications. In this sense, their transitions share long-standing commonalities with British working-class youth, both BAME and white, living in inner-city areas and outer estates (see, *inter alia*, Sewell 1997, Willis 1977, McDowell 2004). Many Manor young people had experienced various forms of school exclusion, while expressions of disliking school were commonplace. At the same time, several young men and women in Manor also wished they had worked harder at school (see also Lloyd 1999):

> **Kandy** [white female, 17]: I hated school, but if I could go back I would behave so much, I'd sit down and do my work.... I used to be naughty all the time – they [teachers] used to say to me, 'Oh, do your work,' and I would say, 'What's the point?'
> **AG**: Why couldn't you see the point of doing your schoolwork back then?
> **Kandy**: Nah, I used to think, well, I'm gonna get a job no matter what, but I was wrong.
> **AG**: What kind of job did you want?
> **Kandy**: I wanted to work in an office, but then I wanted to be a solicitor, but that's nang.[8]

In previously wanting to become a solicitor, Kandy demonstrated high occupational aspirations, as did many of the young people in Manor. Since leaving school, Kandy had applied for several entry-level office jobs, but was unable to obtain such a position because she did not have any GCSE passes at grades A–C. Kandy was NEET for almost two years before getting onto the New Deal for Young People programme when she turned 18.

On leaving school, the majority of young men and women in Manor will be 'going college' by enrolling at a local further education (FE) college as well as obtaining part-time or casual employment within the 'clean' service sector. For these young people, road culture still provides the focal point of their leisure activities. Another post-16 career trajectory is that of 'working on road', whereby a small number of young males will become more involved in the spectacular and hyper-masculine aspects of road life.

Grafting for a living: doing the dirty work

There is a residue of traditional male manual jobs available in London, at least for those males 'in the know'; that is, immersed in the right social networks (Watt 2003). This is borne out in Manor whereby some young men, adherents of the grafter youth subculture, have obtained regular or casual, full-time, paid work as unskilled labourers, forklift truck operators, builders' mates or apprentice electricians on various City and Dockland construction sites. Although the construction workforce has been on a long-term, downward trajectory in London since the early 1970s, it has not experienced the same precipitous decline as manufacturing (GLA Economics 2007).

The grafters are a group of young men, predominantly although not exclusively white, who reside on the low-rise Michaels' Estate. This comprises a core group of six young men – one black, one mixed-parentage and the other four white – but includes up to 10 additional white youths who are attached to the group. This group is aged from 17 to 20 years and is distinguished by its positive attitude to manual labour. With one exception, they are all committed to earning a living through 'grafting' in the construction industry either as labourers or apprentice tradesmen. For such young men, getting and securing a 'proper' manual job is viewed as an important sign of 'manhood' and adulthood (see Johnston *et al.* 2000). Since leaving school, the grafters have 'matured' a great deal; whereas in the past they were involved in petty crime and joyriding around the neighbourhood on stolen mopeds or in 'nicked' cars, now they are on the whole 'law-abiding citizens'. As such, despite economic restructuring, this group of young men still managed to undertake a 'traditional', working-class, masculine, school-to-work transition, as described by Willis (1977).

This transition was aided by the fact that even before leaving school many of the grafters had been used to working on building sites as labourers for cash-in-hand payments. However, the main opportunity for casual cash-in-hand work was obtained through Simon, a fellow Michaels' Estate resident, who came from Nigeria to live in London. By taking advantage of the informalization of low-level service work that has become a key feature of London's changing labour market (Abrams 2002, Smith 2005), Simon was able to operate a small-scale company that was subcontracted to clean office blocks in the City and Docklands outside office hours. In their later school years, aged 14–16, many of the grafters used to work for Simon off and on as cleaners. He would pick up all those young men who were interested in his van at 10 p.m. each night and drop them back home at 6 a.m. the next morning, paying them in cash at the end of each shift.

The grafters obtained paid employment through their extensive social networks of family and friends, as was also found by Lloyd (1999) in his study of young men and the labour market. On leaving school, Sparky (white male, 17) originally secured full-time employment as a labourer on a building site, as a result of his father's contacts in the 'trade'. Within a few months of meeting his girlfriend, Sparky managed to get taken on as an apprentice electrician at his girlfriend's father's company. Hickman (white male, 19) had never been unemployed for more than three weeks in any one period. In the three years since leaving school, he had obtained full-time employment as a carpet fitter, a mate to an air-conditioning installations engineer, a lift engineer's mate and a construction site labourer. Most of his work had been obtained through his uncle, friends and neighbours, or contacts in the local pub. Indeed, the local pubs of East London serve as unofficial job centres – as well as centres of deviant or criminal activity – for members of the wider East London grafter community (Hobbs 1988). While young black people might 'diss' the pub culture of the grafters, when young white males reach school-leaving age, their recreational and leisure sites shift from the 'road' to that of the pubs, where they will also gain access to information about jobs as well as other (legal and illegal) money-making opportunities. In her report on young men's experiences in the labour market during the 1990s, Meadows (2001, p. 6) found that a 'recurring theme in the research has been the findings that social networks remain one of the most important means of finding a job for young people'. Indeed, such informal networks are likely to be of greater importance in relation to construction given increased subcontracting and the growing proportion of self-employment in London's construction workforce (GLA 2006b).

As a young black male (aged 19), Eddie is totally ensconced within grafter culture. Many of Eddie's black peers view him as 'different' (i.e. from the stereotypical perception of what a young black male should be like), in that he dresses differently and talks 'cockney like a white guy who don't hang around with black people'. Eddie himself is aware of the conflict and argues that most of his friends are white because of where he lives (Michaels' Estate) and where he happened to grow up. The Michaels' Estate is a low-rise public housing complex interspersed with small ex-council prefab housing stock, where some of the residents have exercised the 'right to buy'; although ethnically mixed, this estate is still viewed within the neighbourhood as a 'white estate'. Although he attended college briefly, Eddie works in a builder's yard as a forklift driver, and walks about the street (on leaving work) with his 'dusty clothes, builder's boots and newspaper in his back pocket'. In contrast to Eddie, Lazy Boy (white/black African parentage, 19) had never 'had a proper job for more than two weeks'. His friends would obtain labouring opportunities for him on various construction sites through their contacts, but after a few weeks Lazy Boy would get 'fed up' with the 'hard graft' and 'jack in' the job. Eddie's and Lazy Boy's experiences highlight how it was possible for black and mixed-parentage young men to access grafting opportunities as a result of where they lived in Manor, even though the grafting employment networks were dominated by older, white males. Women, however, were excluded; informal working-class job networks in London appear to be largely gender-homogeneous (Watt 2003).

Going to college: in search of clean work

If the youth labour market has dramatically contracted during the last 30 years, young people's participation rate in post-compulsory education has more than doubled, with young BAME people especially likely either to stay on at school or go to college (Cregan 2002). In Manor, most of the young men and women attended FE college as well as working in part-time, service-sector jobs, as in shops or youth work. Young black men like Raymond (black male, 17), Sweet Boy (black male, 17) and Griot (black male, 19) were enrolled in full-time college courses, seeking 'clean' office and hi-tech employment that required 'brain power' as opposed to 'hard graft'. In fact, many of the young, black, male informants in Manor saw manual labour as poorly paid 'dirty work'. 'Clean work', on the other hand, required paper qualifications, so, despite their often unsatisfactory school experiences, most black young men enrolled on full-time college courses.

The young, black and mixed-parentage (and some young, white) females also attended full-time college courses, but were more evenly split between academic and vocational study. While there have been substantial increases in the numbers of young people participating in post-compulsory education, more than one-third of those students enrolled in a full-time college course will fail to complete their studies either as a result of leaving early or because they failed their examinations and/or written assessments (Audit Commission-OFSTED report 1993; cited in Coles 1995, p. 52). During the period of fieldwork, both Raymond and Sweet Boy subsequently failed to complete their studies.

Raymond had learning difficulties and found it difficult to complete his assignments on his college course; his 'messing about' during classes compounded this. He would regularly come into the youth centre in order to get assistance with his written assignments from the youth workers. One evening when Raymond came into the youth centre asking for help, he had a half-written assignment in his hand and continued his dramatic plea for help: 'This is serious [to AG], you got to help me 'cos if I don't do well in this assignment, then they'll probably throw me off the course.' It was clear that, for all his 'messing about', Raymond was in his own way committed to his course of study, but he was struggling academically and did not know how to get the required support at the college. Toward the end of Raymond's first year there, he was suspended for 'fighting' with a fellow student. Even though Raymond was eventually allowed back into college a month later, during the period of his suspension, he fell further behind with his coursework. Raymond's suspension was to have long-term consequences in that, while he managed eventually to pass the course, he did not obtain enough credits to proceed onto the next (more advanced) level course. Sweet Boy was 'kicked-off' his college course due to poor attendance and his failure to submit any coursework. Raymond and Sweet Boy were not the only young, black males who failed to complete their college studies. For a variety of different reasons, all of the young men and some of the young women would eventually drop out and fail to complete their courses.

At the same time as attending college, Sweet Boy obtained a part-time job at the youth club as a junior play/youth leader. Initially, Sweet Boy showed great enthusiasm for his newly acquired position and was an enthusiastic and diligent worker. A few months later, however, he was starting to turn up late for work or not bother to turn up at all, while at work he seemed to be lethargic and uninterested. Less than six months after he was employed at the youth club, Sweet Boy decided to quit his job (before the decision could be taken out of his hands, as the senior youth worker was tiring of Sweet Boy's antics), and set about finding full-time employment. After a short spell of NEET, Sweet Boy found work as a commission-only, door-to-door sales agent for an electricity company, although he soon gave up this job and made tentative steps back into the world of part-time play work. That Sweet Boy's post-16 'cyclical' school-to-work history never seemed to 'move toward more secure, rewarding employment' mirrors the findings of MacDonald *et al.* (2005, p. 881).

Raymond (who also did paid play work), Sweet Boy and Ayesha (who was a part-time dance tutor at the youth club while also attending college) began their play and/or youth work 'careers' as young volunteers before becoming junior workers in the Manor youth club. Some young men and women in Manor saw youth and play work as a 'cushy number' compared to the 'real world' of work. However, genuine career progression within these fields for Raymond and the others would necessitate obtaining higher-level qualifications.

Bradley (2005) has rightly argued that the discourse of 'winners and losers' is both pervasive and ideological in relation to thinking about how young people are positioned within the new economy. While we recognize the limitations of such a discourse, it is also the case that during the period of fieldwork two young black females did successfully complete their college courses, which facilitated entry to professional-managerial career paths. Ayesha (aged 17), for example, had a long-standing interest in dancing and enrolled on a full-time BTEC Diploma in Performing Arts and eventually went on to become a professional dancer, performing in West End shows after several years of study.

Road culture and working on road

The term 'road', as opposed to 'street', culture has been used throughout this paper in recognition of the young people's own definition of their subculture as 'being on road' or as 'living on road'. There is a subtle distinction between the latter two, since whereas the majority of young people might talk of 'being on road' and 'catching joke' with their friends or looking to make 'links', it is only those young people involved in 'badness' who are referred to as 'living on road'. Badness, as defined by the young people themselves, refers to a social world characterized by 'spectacular', hyper-aggressive/hyper-masculine modes of behaviour, incorporating violent and petty crime, fraud or personal identity theft, and low-level drug dealing (see Gunter 2008 for a detailed discussion of badness in Manor).

While the majority of the young people can be viewed as voracious but judicious consumers of road cultural life, for a small minority of young men 'life pon road' consumes most aspects of their day-to-day lives. Road culture in Manor can be viewed as a continuum, where occupying the centre ground are the vast majority of non-spectacular young people, with a small minority of young males or 'rude boys' – who immerse themselves in the world of 'badness' – taking up the extreme margins. However, at the same time, there is also fluidity between the centre ground and the margins. Some young black males (like Raymond and Sweet Boy) occasionally dip in and out of 'badness' as and when they see fit or, more to the point, when a particularly good opportunity arises for them to make some 'easy money'.

The 'badness' that takes place within Manor and its surrounds is largely perpetuated by a small number of young men in crews,[9] with the most prominent being the Arms House Crew, who have built up their 'reps' over a number of years. The Arms House Crew are a loose collective of eight young black males (but including up to another 11 individuals), aged 17–21 years, who live around the notoriously 'rough' Arms House area of Manor. This area comprises a small number of high-rise tower blocks interspersed with privately owned terraced housing, and it is viewed locally as both more 'rough' and more 'black'. As Watt (2006, p. 788) argues, a nuanced 'geography of roughness', one largely invisible to outsiders, operates *within* London's marginal spaces.

The young males in Manor who were involved in 'badness' would not refer to themselves as 'criminals'; rather, they viewed 'living on road' as a form of work (see Johnston *et al.* 2000, MacDonald and Shildrick 2007) that normally involves attempting to earn money from such illegal activities as street robbery, low-level drug dealing, fraud or 'robbing-to-order'.[10] 'Working on road' was interspersed with periods of benefit claiming, but also formal employment for some members of the Arms House Crew. Nathaniel [black male, 18], for example, lived at home with his mother and younger brother, and had worked off and on (through his aunt's contacts) in a variety of entry-level, office-based jobs in the City and a local authority housing department. Nathaniel was interested in 'living on road' because he felt it was the only way (other than perhaps youth work) that he could make money without having to be 'bored' or put up with 'bullshit' from 'chiefs in suits'. Comments from other crew members about not wanting a 'shit-paying job' or to be bossed about by some 'racist idiot' reflect their emphasis on maintaining a masculine form of 'respect' (Bourgois 1995), as well as refusal to put up with everyday racism. Contemporary post-industrial workplaces represent an alien world for many young people in Manor, since 'street culture is in direct contradiction to the humble, obedient modes of subservient social interaction that are essential for upward mobility in high-rise office jobs' (Bourgois 1995, p. 142).

Conclusion

Drawing on research and interview data from a larger ethnographic youth study undertaken in one deprived East London neighbourhood, this paper has outlined three divergent (yet similarly restrictive) post-16 career paths for young males; it has also referred, albeit in less detail, to the young female informants' post-16 experiences. No one single transition predominated in Manor, as MacDonald *et al.* (2001) also found in Teesside's marginal spaces. The young male and female informants did exercise a degree of agency with regards to their school-to-work transitions. Such agency and 'choices' were mediated through ethnicity, gender, neighbourhood networks, and the road and grafter subcultures. Their transitions were shaped, albeit not mechanistically determined, by recent economic restructuring and the growth of the new economy, in addition to long-standing, working-class survival tactics in East London whereby 'getting by' can mean resorting to informal and/or illegal means as a supplement, or even alternative, to formal employment (Hobbs 1988, Hood and Joyce 1999).

Like other marginal zones in London, Manor is not a US-style 'jobless ghetto' (Buck 2002, Wacquant 2008). At the same time, obtaining entry-level jobs can be difficult, as some of the young people's recurring NEET experiences testify. Having left school with few or no qualifications, the young people in Manor had to navigate their way through the city's new economy, which could, at best, offer them low-paid employment within various service industries or else manual jobs within construction. Relying upon their low-level educational qualifications *alone* would by no means guarantee entry to employment. It is striking how many of the young informants, both black and white, accessed jobs through drawing upon whatever social capital they possessed in the form of relatives and acquaintances inside workplaces 'speaking for them'.

The relative buoyancy of London's construction industry means that a well-trodden transition is still available to young males who possess a positive attitude to dirty, hard graft, and who can also access key neighbourhood employment networks and subculture. Grafter culture demonstrates continuities with traditional 'learning to labour', masculine, working-class transitions (Willis 1977) as well as East London particularities of 'ducking and diving' (Hobbs 1988). The grafters remain connected to the well-trodden – albeit diminishing and increasingly insecure – employment pathways available within construction. The major difference, however, between the 1970s and 2000s is that the employment base of grafter culture in London is largely restricted to what amounts to the niche construction industry, since its other, larger pole, manufacturing, has so contracted. Although white-dominated, grafter culture is not racially exclusive, since young, black men, such as Eddie, can adopt its valorization of 'hard graft', while older, black men like Simon employ white youths in the bargain-basement end of labour subcontracting in the cleaning industry. At the same time, as Watt (2003, p. 1785) argues, 'those who [are] either outside or on the margins of the social networks connected to job information, because of ethnicity or social isolation, [are] in a far weaker labour market position'. The dominance of grafting networks by older, white, working-class males means that young black men in Manor, as well as young women per se, are much more likely to be 'out of the loop' when word-of-mouth job opportunities are passed around.

In contrast to the grafters, most of the black young people and some of the young white women sought to go to college, so that they might one day obtain better-paid, 'clean', service-sector jobs. Dirt and cleanliness are culturally encoded via the social hierarchies of paid work (Wolkowitz 2007). The fact, therefore, that most young black men in Manor 'diss' grafter culture as being 'dirty work' and say that they prefer 'clean work' in services and offices can be seen to represent an embrace of the new economy with its middle-class image as opposed to the residues of traditional, working-class, manual employment. Such a preference is also prefigured in valorizing aspects of road culture, notably consumption and dress, which militate against having a 'dirty' appearance. The mundane reality of the new economy is that the service-sector jobs that the young men and women can realistically obtain, given their limited educational qualifications, are routine, subservient, low-paid and often insecure (McDowell 2004, Bradley 2005).

While the majority of young black males in Manor – who will enrol in full-time college courses on leaving school at age 16 – flirt with the style and aesthetics of badness, they nonetheless buy into mainstream discourses about social inclusion, equality of opportunity and hyper-consumption as propagated by official government agencies, the media and cultural industries. However, the subtext to these messages is that 'success' is only available to those men and women who fully participate in post-16 education and training. Despite appealing to many young, black people because it offered the possibility of accessing better-paid 'clean work', going to college is fraught with potential pitfalls, including the risk of replicating their often unsatisfactory school experiences; as we saw, most eventually dropped out of college. In order to thrive in the alien worlds of formal education and service employment, they would have somehow to disengage from the familiar road culture and its attendant bodily 'habitus' of speech and style (Bourdieu 1990). If racial discrimination against BAME groups in London is also factored in (Fieldhouse 1998), one can appreciate how young black people in Manor in particular are making 'choices' within tightly circumscribed boundaries.

In contrast, by rejecting the official discourses of 'equality of opportunity', the Arm's House Crew follow parallel paths to other black Atlantic (and Latino) young males of 'low social status', in wanting to maintain respect and earn a living on *their* terms (Anderson 1990, Bourgois 1995). Within this context, it is clear why some young black men in Manor choose to deepen their involvement in the familiarities of road culture and the attendant risks associated with 'working on road', risks further compounded by the fact that young black men are, in comparison to other ethnic groupings, more likely to be targeted by the police and other authorities, and once caught up within the criminal justice process, are punished more harshly (see Crown Prosecution Service 2003).

Notes

1. Pseudonyms are used throughout the paper for neighbourhood place names and respondents' names.
2. According to the 2001 Census, there was a significant minority of Asian families living in Manor; however, the field researcher (AG) was unable to identify any groups of Asian young people for inclusion in the study. This could be explained by the fact that while many of the informants attended (or had attended) school with Asian young people, they did not 'hang out' socially with them.
3. In 'catching joke', young people relay humorous stories and situations back to each other, talk about girls or boys, and generally 'diss' (name-calling/mickey taking) each other.
4. 'Links' or 'link-ups': sexual liaisons between young men and young women – more than just friends but less than girl/boyfriends.
5. To 'kotch' is to sit down and relax or stay in one place, as opposed to 'passing through' or being 'on a mission' when the young person concerned is busy and on the move –perhaps because they have places to go or other people to see.

6. To 'pass through'; here the young persons concerned are not looking to 'hang out' – they have just briefly stopped by, maybe to see someone or pick something up (money, a message, clothes, etc.), before going on their way again.
7. The proportion of women employed in construction in London was the lowest of all industry sectors in 2003; furthermore, it has hardly increased since the early 1980s despite a substantial overall increase in the percentage of female workers (GLA 2006a).
8. 'Nang' is a street term for 'rubbish, crap or stupid'.
9. In using the term 'crews' as opposed to 'gangs', the authors concur with Hallsworth and Young's (2008) critique of the growing media and academic preoccupation with the UK youth gang phenomenon. Hallsworth and Young note that street-based interpersonal youth violence is not always reducible to the 'gang'; rather there are often a number of complex local factors that need to be taken into account (see Gunter 2008).
10. In 'robbing-to-order', a fence or middleman asks a rude boy or out-there-boy to steal a particular item or items, such as car alloy wheels, car stereos, laptop computers, mobile phones, or designer clothes.

References

Abrams, F., 2002. *Below the breadline: living on the minimum wage.* London: Profile Books.

Anderson, E., 1990. *Streetwise.* Chicago: University of Chicago Press.

Bourdieu, P., 1990. *The logic of practice.* Stanford, CA: Stanford University Press.

Bourgois, P., 1995. *In search of respect: selling crack in el bario.* Cambridge: Cambridge University Press.

Bradley, H., 2005. Winners and losers: young people in the 'new economy'. *In*: H. Bradley and J van Hoof, eds. *Young people in Europe: labour markets and citizenship.* Bristol: Policy Press, 99–113.

Buck N., Gordon, I., Hall, P., Harloe, M., and Kleinman, M., 2002. *Working capital: life and labour in contemporary London.* London: Routledge.

Cohen, P., 1996. All white on the night: narratives of nativism on the Isle of Dogs. *In*: T. Butler and M. Rustin, eds. *Rising in the East: the regeneration of East London.* London: Lawrence & Wishart, 170–196.

Cohen, P. and Ainley, P., 2000. In the country of the blind? Youth studies and cultural studies in Britain. *Journal of youth studies*, 3 (1), 79–95.

Coles, B., 1995. *Youth and social policy.* London: UCL Press.

Cregan, C., 2002. Are things really getting better? The labour market experience of black and female youth at the start of the century. *Capital and class*, 77, 23–52.

Crown Prosecution Service, 2003. *Race for justice: a review of Crown Prosecution Service decision making for possible racial bias at each stage of the prosecution process.* London: Crown Prosecution Service.

Fieldhouse, E.A., 1998. Ethnic minority unemployment and spatial mismatch: the case of London. *Urban studies*, 39, 1569–1596.

Gilroy, P., 1993. *The Black Atlantic: modernity and double consciousness.* London: Verso.

GLA Economics, 2006a. *Women at work – looking ahead* (Working Paper 16). London: Greater London Authority.

GLA Economics, 2006b. *Laying the foundations: London's construction industry.* London: Greater London Authority.

GLA Economics, 2007. *An analysis of London's employment by sector* (Working Paper 24). London: Greater London Authority.

Gunter, A., 2008. Growing up bad: black youth, 'road' culture and badness in an East London neighbourhood. *Crime, media, culture*, 4(3), 349-365.

Gunter, A., 2009, forthcoming. *Growing up bad: road culture, badness and black youth transitions in an East London neighbourhood.* London: Tufnell Press.

Hallsworth, S. and Young, T., 2008. Gang talk and gang talkers: a critique. *Crime, media, culture*, 4 (2), 175–195.

Hamnett, C., 2003. *Unequal city: London in the global arena.* London: Routledge.

Hobbs, D., 1988. *Doing the business: entrepreneurship, detectives and the working class in the East End of London.* Oxford: Oxford University Press.

Hood, R. and Joyce, K., 1999. Three generations: oral testimonies on crime and social change in London's East End. *British journal of criminology*, 39 (1), 136–160.
Johnston, L., Macdonald, R., Mason, P., Ridley, L. and Webster, C., 2000. *Snakes and ladders: young people, transitions and social exclusion*. Bristol: Joseph Rowntree Foundation/Policy Press.
Lloyd, T., 1999. *Young men, the job market and gendered work*. York: Joseph Rowntree Foundation/York Publishing Services.
LDA (London Development Agency), 2006. *Targeting worklessness in London – socio-economic analysis* (Technical Annex). London: London Development Agency.
MacDonald, R., Mason, P., Shildrick, T., Webster, C., Johnston, L., and Ridley, L., 2001. Snakes and ladders: in defence of youth transition. *Sociological research online*, 5 (4), www.socresonline.org.uk/5/4/macdonald.html [Accessed 12 January 2009].
MacDonald, R., Shildrick, T., Webster, C., and Simpson, D., 2005. Growing up in poor neighbourhoods: the significance of class and place in the extended transitions of 'socially excluded' young adults. *Sociology*, 39 (5), 873–891.
MacDonald, R., and Shildrick, T., 2007. Street corner society: leisure careers, youth (sub)culture and social exclusion. *Leisure studies*, 26(3), 339–355.
McDowell, L., 2004. *Redundant masculinities? Employment change and white working class youth*. Oxford: Blackwell.
Meadows, P., 2001. *Young men on the margins: an overview report*. York: Joseph Rowntree Foundation/York Publishing Services.
Nayak, A., 2003. *Race, place and globalization: youth cultures in a changing world*. Oxford: Berg.
ODPM, 2004. *Index of multiple deprivation*. London: Office for the Deputy Prime Minister.
PACEC (Public and Corporate Economic Consultants), 2003. *Understanding London's sub-regional economies*. London: London Development Agency.
Research as Evidence, 2007. *What works in preventing and re-engaging young people NEET in London*. London: Greater London Authority.
Reynolds, T., 2007. Friendship networks, social capital and ethnic identity: researching the perspectives of Caribbean young people in Britain. *Journal of youth studies*, 10(4), 383–398.
Roberts, K., 1995. *Youth and employment in modern Britain*. Oxford: Oxford University Press.
Sewell, T., 1997. *Black masculinities and schooling: how black boys survive modern schooling*. Stoke-on-Trent: Trentham Books.
Shildrick, T. and MacDonald, R., 2007. In defence of subculture: young people, leisure and social divisions. *Journal of youth studies*, 9 (2), 125–140.
Smith, D.M., 2005. *On the margins of inclusion: changing labour markets and social exclusion in London*. Bristol: Policy Press.
Syrett, S. and North, D., 2008. *Renewing neighbourhoods: work, enterprise and governance*. Bristol: Policy Press.
Wacquant, L., 2008. *Urban outcasts: a comparative sociology of advanced marginality*. Cambridge: Polity Press.
Watt, P., 2003. Urban marginality and economic restructuring: local authority tenants and employment in an inner London borough. *Urban studies*, 40 (9), 1769–1789.
Watt, P., 2006. Respectability, roughness and 'race': neighbourhood place images and the making of working-class social distinctions in London. *International journal of urban and regional research*, 30 (4), 776–797.
Watt, P. and Stenson, K., 1998. The street: it's a bit dodgy around there: safety, danger, ethnicity and young people's use of public space. *In*: T. Skelton and G. Valentine, eds. *Cool places: geographies of youth cultures*. London: Routledge, 299–265.
Willis, P., 1977. *Learning to labour: how working class kids get working class jobs*. Farnborough: Gower.
Wolkowitz, C., 2007. Linguistic leakiness or really dirty? Dirt in social theory. *In*: B. Campkin and R. Cox, eds. *Dirt: new geographies of cleanliness and contamination*. London: I.B. Tauris, 15–24.

From 'inheritance' to individualization: disembedding working-class youth transitions in post-Soviet Russia

Charlie Walker

Russian and Eurasian Studies Centre and CEELBAS, St Antony's College, University of Oxford, Oxford, UK

Despite the impoverishment of prospects for those employed in the industrial and agricultural sectors in post-Soviet Russia, young people in vocational education colleges continue to be trained for 'poor work' in traditional large-scale enterprises. This article draws upon qualitative, case-study research in exploring young people's subjective orientations to a route to adulthood that is at once available and yet unviable, as well as their orientations to new forms of education and service sector employment. The article highlights the disjuncture which has emerged between the collectivist, class-based identities and modalities young people construct around transitions into initial vocational education and training (IVET) colleges and the individualized, choice-based narratives they use to describe experiences of later transitions into work. This shift from 'inheritance' to 'individualization' mirrors that among working-class youth elsewhere in the world, for whom the principal dimension of 'reflexivity' in the late-modern context has been the individualized attribution of blame for 'wrong choices'.

Introduction

> There's nothing to like about working there. They don't pay you, they pay you nothing, neither workers nor students training there. What's the point of staying at your workplace? It's just for people who've got nowhere to go – they just work for kopeks (pennies) year after year. (Sergey, metal worker, 18)

In most Western industrialized societies, young people leaving school with few academic qualifications face very different prospects from those of their parents' generation, as processes of deindustrialization and the emergence of globalized, flexible labour markets have replaced traditional working-class jobs with feminized and hyphenated forms of service sector employment. While a new policy emphasis on educational participation has apparently offered such young people opportunities to 'reinvent' themselves, the reality of growing up 'working class' has often been one of growing insecurity and a polarization of life chances *vis-à-vis* the wider population (MacDonald and Marsh 2005). In post-Soviet Russia, the unravelling of working-class routes to adulthood has taken a somewhat different form, resulting not from the gradual economic shift which has taken place in most Western societies, but from the catastrophic collapse of a state-led economic system. The collapse of this system, which precipitated what has been described as the worst recession in human history (Clarke 1999, p. 1), led not to widespread unemployment, but to an impoverishment of prospects for those employed in the industrial and agricultural sectors, in which poverty wages, unsafe working conditions and extended periods of unpaid leave continue to be the norm for many (Yaroshenko *et al.* 2006, p. 134). Despite this, however, Russia's largely unreformed initial vocational education and training (IVET) system remains heavily integrated into the manufacturing and production sectors, and continues to train young people for 'poor work' in large-scale traditional enterprises (Walker 2006). In this context, traditional routes to adulthood continue to be available to working-class youth in Russia, while at the same time being entirely unviable. This article addresses the ways in which young people graduating from IVET colleges in Ul'yanovsk – an industrialized province in Russia's Volga region – experience these 'transitions to nowhere', and how the contradiction it poses is reflected in their biographical narratives and identity construction.

The principal theoretical concern of the article is to examine the ways in which contemporary theories regarding the 'individualization' and 'destandardization' of the life course (Giddens 1991, Beck 1992, Beck and Beck-Gernsheim 1995) might apply to the lives of 'working-class kids' in provincial Russia. While these ideas have enjoyed wide currency in the sociology of youth for a number of years, studies of young people with differing social characteristics (along the lines of class, gender, ethnicity and place) and in a range of different cultural and institutional contexts, have often found them to be inadequate, or at least problematic, conceptual tools. Nilsen and Brannen (2002, p. 35), for example, regard the notion that late modernity has witnessed a transition from 'normal' to 'choice' biographies (Beck 1992, Beck and Beck-Gernsheim 1995) as too simplistic, pointing instead to a duality of experimental and traditional orientations in the life plans of young people in several European countries. Similarly, Thomson and Holland (2002, p. 339) argue that, while processes of detraditionalization imply a weakening of the determining influence of gender, 'in practice, the pulls of tradition still operate, and are most acutely felt by young women who are more willing to accommodate their careers with family demands than are young men.' The ability of late modernity to 'disembed' traditional aspects of social identity and the cultural scripts that accompany them is further questioned by MacDonald and Marsh (2005, p. 211). Their research, exploring the lives of working-class youth in a 'socially excluded' region of north-east England, points to the class cultural scripts which appear still to shape their respondents' ways of coping with the loss of work and the variety of local deprivations that accompany this. Indeed, the capacity of late modernity not to disembed, but to *re*-embed what Beck calls 'industrial society ways of life' (Beck 1994, p. 13) is echoed in studies of young people growing up in the post-socialist countries of Eastern Europe. Commenting on research among young people in Serbia, for example, Tomanović and Ignjatović (2006, p. 272) argue that, in contrast to trends identified in Western societies, 'retraditionalization is present in all domains of private and family life' (see also Wallace 1995, Glendinning *et al.* 2004).

The notion of a re-embedding of individuals not into 'abstract systems' and 'markets' (Giddens 1991, p. 137), but into more traditional, even pre-modern forms of socio-cultural integration, is fully supported by the research upon which the present article is based. As I explore elsewhere (Walker forthcoming), the ways in which graduates of IVET colleges in Ul'yanovsk responded to 'transitions to nowhere' pointed not to the pushing back of individuals onto their own resources, but to a deepening of traditional forms of dependency and interdependency rooted in family, kinship and locality. Attempts to migrate to other cities, for example, or to find alternative forms of employment, were negotiated primarily through whatever resources were available to the respondents within their informal networks, rather than through individual negotiation of the labour and housing markets or any intermediary systems connected to them. To a large extent, this is reflective of the wider exclusionary processes which have taken place across many post-socialist countries in the process of economic 'transition'. As old institutional structures and forms of state provision have been dismantled, the neo-liberal, largely market-based forms of social organization which have replaced them have rarely functioned in the classical, open manner intended by the architects of reform. Rather, people have had to learn to live with and negotiate markets that are by turns undeveloped, inaccessible, corrupt or unregulated (Stenning 2008), and dealing with these has often meant a greater reliance on close-knit, horizontal networks of social ties (Rose 1998), not least for young people. In this context, the notion of a choice-making, individualized subject who is integrated into society through markets, abstract systems and formal institutions appears difficult to uphold.

In other respects, however, the notions of individual choice and responsibility have become central to young people's transitions to adulthood in Russia, and were pervasive in the subjectivities and narratives of IVET students in Ul'yanovsk. While the respondents' attempts to negotiate different aspects of their transitions to adulthood continued to be shaped by very localized resources and traditional dependencies, the ways in which they thought about and described past, present and future possibilities for working careers was indicative of the disembedding of collectively experienced forms of identity suggested by theorists of reflexive modernity. Upon graduating from IVET colleges, the young people in the research were confronted simultaneously by the abject conditions and prospects of poor work in industrial enterprises and by the emergence of a range of new opportunities in service sector employment and the higher education system. The latter, which has opened up the possibility of attending university to young people who had traditionally left the education system at the earliest opportunity, has been particularly transformative in defining the types of opportunities young people believe to be open to them. The fact that the emergence of these pathways – which appear to offer the prospect of highly desirable careers in fashionable professions such as management and marketing – has coincided with the impoverishment of the educational route taken by the respondents was starkly reflected in the narratives of choice they used to describe their transitions. As they were thrust into an environment that forced them to construct individual routes through emerging educational and labour market structures, identities rooted in older, more collective forms of transition became contradictory and anachronistic, such that the construction of new pathways served to disembed the 'sense' of their prior choices, and the narratives of identity that had been underpinned by them. In order to illuminate this contradiction, and the process of individualization engendered by it, it is necessary to go back to the ways in which identities were constructed among the respondents as they experienced earlier transitions into and through IVET colleges, and to revisit a theory of youth cultural identity developed by Phil Cohen.

Cohen's theory of 'reproduction codes' (1997), like Willis' 'counter-school culture' (1977), centred on the ways in which processes of formal and informal learning acted as focal points in the construction of young people's cultural biographies and identities. These codes – 'apprenticeship', 'inheritance', 'vocation' and 'career' – expressed the ways in which class relations were subjectively experienced and symbolically represented in both working-class and middle-class cultures. The way the notion of skill is subjectively constructed in working-class culture, for example, is as a 'birthright' or a 'legacy': 'not so much a socially achieved practice as an inherent property' (Cohen 1997, p. 205). As such, while middle-class youth transitions revolved around the codes of 'vocation' and 'career', Cohen saw growing-up working class as being 'an apprenticeship to ... an inheritance – a patrimony of skill entailed in the body and its techniques, forging a quasi-congenital link between origins and destinies' (p. 205). While young men underwent an induction into traditions of manual skill on the shop floor, working-class young women's apprenticeships entailed the acquisition of skills which centred on, and produced their subordination within, the domestic sphere (p. 233). Meanwhile, the family, peer groups, and locality were all important transmitters of and contexts for these class-cultural apprenticeships. What Cohen wanted to emphasize in constructing this model was what he saw as the weakening of old markers of working-class identity over the course of the 1980s, which had resulted both from the disappearance of traditional routes into work and from the formalized training schemes which sought to replace them. In the latter, Cohen saw an attempt to replace traditional working-class definitions of skill with a formalized system rooted in the individualist ethos of Thatcherism, such that the grids of 'inheritance' and 'apprenticeship' were being weakened and pulled apart by the imposition of the 'career' code.

In many respects, Cohen's examination of working-class lives under the new vocationalism identifies what more recent literatures would describe as a process of individualization: a disembedding of class modalities which, in the absence of traditional forms of employment, can no longer act as the cultural scripts they had once been. MacDonald and Marsh (2005, p. 212) describe a similar situation in Teesside. While they find that traditional working-class identities and ways of life continue to pervade their conversations with young people, they also find that 'deindustrialization has progressively stripped away the economic structures in which ... working-class cultural tastes and outlooks ... "worked" and made sense.' More broadly, these studies of working-class youth speak to wider debates regarding changes in the nature of employment in Western societies, and the (in)ability of the new world of work to support the coherent, often class-based identities and life narratives that characterized working lives in the past (Sennett 1998, Bauman 2005). It is with the post-socialist experience of this disjuncture – between traditional forms of identity and biographical narrative, on the one hand, and the objective conditions to support them, on the other hand – that this article is concerned.

Parallels between the experience of the Soviet working class and its British counterpart cannot, of course, be made without qualification. The formal existence of a 'workers' state', for example, precluded the existence of an oppositional labour politics in the USSR, such that the bases of working-class identity were in one respect fundamentally different. Nevertheless, what we know about patterns and processes of class reproduction in the Soviet Union (although we lack Soviet equivalents to Willis's ethnography) indicates much commonality of experience. Indeed, if anything, the extent to which labour market transitions among working-class youth replicated those of their parents and previous generations was even greater, with the tendency for family work biographies to take place through the same professions and in the same factories epitomized by the official celebration of 'worker dynasties' (Tkach 2003) and the subjective orientation of workers to the enterprise as a 'second home' (Clarke 1999, p. 16). As regards the post-Soviet context, the dislocations of economic restructuring that are defining the experience of the working class in Western societies have been more pronounced. Indeed, the situation faced by young people graduating from IVET colleges in Ul'yanovsk places the notion of a non-congruity between old forms of identity and new economic realities into stark relief, precisely because it engenders a disjuncture that is experienced and reflected not simply across generations, but within individual biographies. As will be explored in the first section of the article, the objective institutional framework provided by Russia's IVET system and the enterprises to which it is connected combines with and reinforces the respondents' subjective identifications with peers, locality, and forms of manual skill, in the production of a transition that continues, *up to a point*, to be experienced as an 'apprenticeship' to an 'inheritance'. As such, the realities of 'transitions to nowhere' are experienced by the respondents as an undermining of what had hitherto been relatively straightforward transitions characterized by well-formed notions of labour market identities and positions. As will be explored in the second part of the article, while the new higher education system holds out opportunities for IVET graduates to 're-invent themselves' (Walkerdine *et al.* 2001), many respondents experience this disembedding of a collective identity – a 'normal biography' – as a more negative form of individualization, which consists primarily in the self-attribution of failure for 'wrong choices' or 'choices not made' (Beck 1992, p. 135). Shaped in the context of the wider denigration of working-class identities and ways of life in post-socialism (Stenning 2005, Kideckel 2008), this form of reflexivity – what Giddens (1991) describes as the loss of 'ontological security' – may be seen as constituting the principal dimension of the 'choice biography' for working-class youth in post-Soviet Russia.

The study

The article draws upon qualitative, case-study research carried out in Ul'yanovsk between March and October 2004. Although representativeness was a not a criterion for the study, the choice of Ul'yanovsk was partly based on its largely unexceptional nature in terms of socio-economic indicators. Levels of unemployment, urbanization and wages, for example, are close to the national average (Goskomstat 2005). A further reason for the choice of Ul'yanovsk as the basis of a study focusing on working-class youth was that it is a developed industrial region, in which, in contrast to more service-oriented commercial-financial hubs such as nearby Samara and Kazan, large-scale manufacturing and agricultural enterprises dominate the local economy. As elsewhere in Russia, Ul'yanovsk's industrial enterprises coped with the collapse of the Soviet economy in the early 1990s not by shedding labour, but by reducing working hours and wages (Schwartz 2003). In this context, while open unemployment remained low, enforced periods of 'administrative leave' and the delay or non-payment of already shrunken wage packets became as widespread as more 'normal' forms of exploitation such as low-rate piecework. Despite the upturn in Russia's economy from the late 1990s, all of these problems continued to be evident in the enterprises offering employment to the young people in the research.

As regards the colleges in which the respondents were or had been studying, while there have been attempts to reform the IVET sector since the late 1990s (see Walker 2006), these were largely unreconstructed versions of their former Soviet selves, with most remaining attached to a given 'base enterprise', regardless of the latter's (mis-)fortunes.

The core of the case study consisted of 96 in-depth, semi-structured interviews with final-year students (58) and recent graduates (38) of nine IVET colleges. The colleges were chosen for the variety of subjects they taught, the range of relationships they shared with industry, and their gender profiles (including both single-sex and mixed colleges), while respondents themselves were identified through college staff and snowballing from existing respondents. Like IVET students elsewhere in Russia, the young people in the research were primarily from manual worker and agricultural backgrounds in which parents had obtained similar types of (vocational) education. In what follows all names have been altered to preserve respondents' anonymity. The research adopted an holistic approach to youth transitions (Coles 1995), which was intended to shed light on the types of structural barriers which graduates of IVET colleges faced across different transitional 'strands' (in work, education, family and housing), as well as the resources (social, cultural and material) available to them with which to negotiate these. As such, the research set out to explore the ways in which a range of social inequalities, in particular those rooted in class, place and gender, both underpinned, and were reproduced through, young people's transitions. Although not longitudinal, the study was able to produce a 'longer view' on patterns of transition, both through a comparison of the experiences of final year students and recent graduates, and through the adoption of a biographical, 'life-story' approach (Goodson and Sikes 2001). The retrospective dimension provided by the latter forms the basis of the following section.

An 'apprenticeship' to an 'inheritance': transitions through IVET education

Despite the overwhelmingly low regard in which IVET colleges have always been held by the wider population in Russia (Matthews 1982, pp. 87–88), the majority of the respondents gave entirely positive accounts of their joining the IVET system, particularly when comparing this with their experiences at secondary school. Most had clearly gravitated away from the 'educational exchange' (of subservience for qualifications) some time before the end of the ninth grade, at which point pupils must decide whether to continue in the mainstream secondary school system. While some spoke of an active rejection of school followed by a history of troublemaking, others reported a gradual resignation to the fact that they felt bound to be unsuccessful in this environment:

> I just used to skive off all the time at school ... the teachers nearly cried for joy when I left. (Airat, metal worker, 17)

> I got all '3's ['C's/'D's] at school, I didn't take it that seriously ... I mean, I took it seriously at first, but then the teachers started to look at me differently, started to give me '3's all the time. Then I stopped trying. (Olga, cook, 18)

However, while negative experiences in compulsory education led the majority to complain of having 'had enough' of school, this was by no means a rejection of formal education per se. Rather, this drift away from the academic track was invariably accompanied by an identification with the type of manual skills that would be taught in IVET colleges, or as it was most often put, with 'technology' (*tekhnika*). For many, this differentiation of manual from mental labour was articulated as a 'natural' affinity with technical work, often rooted in childhood experiences and life outside school:

> I like fixing machines, working with cars ... ages ago, when I was just 14, I fixed up an old motorbike with my dad, it's my own motorbike. I just enjoy it. (Anton, metal worker, 18)

> I've always wanted to do something connected with the forest, I don't know, with nature ... maybe it's something inside me, I can't explain it. (Sergey, forester, 20)

For others, it was positive experiences within the education system that had been instrumental in fostering and confirming such dispositions. Some recounted how they had welcomed and been influenced by the introduction of manually based subjects in school:

> I love sewing, I enjoy it ... I've been studying it now for five years ... when we started technology classes in school, I immediately enjoyed sewing, and then came here after the ninth class. (Katya, sewing machinist, 18)

Others mentioned the important role played by careers advice in shaping their choices:

> Yes, in school ... they came into lessons, talked about which professions there were, about what you could do ... They did tests ... about whether you would be better working with nature, with technology, or with people ... well, I'm a 'technical person'. (Denis, machine operator, 20)

Consequently, in contrast to school, the experience of learning in IVET colleges was described as a positive one by most, a 'confirmation' of what were constructed as 'natural' dispositions:

> It's easier to study here, for me, because it's technical education, whereas in school it was more maths, that sort of thing. I mean, it's not easy here either, but all the same, it's more technical so I just like it more. (Vasilii, metal worker, 18)

Alongside the subjective logic of a 'natural affinity' with technical work, choosing to study in IVET colleges also had a clear instrumental rationale stemming from the immediate currency of vocational qualifications on the labour market, and a desire, or often a need, to make transitions into work at the earliest opportunity. In this context, the respondents' colleges provided education which was 'useful', and 'worth' studying for, while for many, entering the IVET system itself was a marker of 'adult' status:

> Here, I mean, I'm getting a trade ... so of course it's more interesting than sitting in school and doing maths tests. (Edik, machine worker, 19)

> Here ... you're already a worker ... someone who's getting a profession, an adult. It's like, more serious. In school you're still children. (Nikolai, mechanic, 19)

Despite this active appropriation of the internal 'logic' of studying in IVET colleges by the majority, a small number of respondents reported that they had aspired to stay on at school and subsequently enter a more prestigious establishment offering secondary rather than initial vocational education. However, the prospect of remaining a full-time student for a further 3 years, and doing so within a fee-based college, made this an unrealistic prospect for most:

> **R:** I wanted to go to the *tekhnikum* [secondary vocational college], but my friends all came here, and I decided to do the same. My mum said, 'Go on, your brother studied there, try and get your builder's trade there.'
> **I:** Did you rethink because of your friends, or because it was paid-for there, and free here?
> **R:** Yes, it was because of the money. (Valerii, builder, 17)

As this example suggests, calculations regarding the costs of secondary vocational education, alongside the overall logic of the IVET route, for some went hand in hand with more socially and culturally embedded identifications of why IVET colleges 'felt right' for them. Especially among the young men in the research, narratives of educational choices often threw up strong associations between different educational establishments and particular, 'other' social groupings:

> I don't know why I liked it more here, I suppose just how it usually happens – you go into a place, you start there and just think, 'This is for me', it's just a feeling . . . I mean, I had a look at the automobile *tekhnikum* but, when I went there, I didn't know about not wearing a tracksuit, so I arrived at the exam and they just escorted me out: 'Here we wear trousers and shirts' [pompously intoned]. (Evgeny, metal worker, 19)

The role played by social identifications such as these was further apparent in the way the respondents described their entrance to specific colleges. According to a recent policy document, young people would make economically rational choices about which colleges to study at on the basis of the links they possessed with particular enterprises (Lebedev 2001, p. 18). In reality, choices were more often hectic, last-minute decisions based on where their friends were going or where either friends or relatives had been previously:

> I don't know, I suppose the lads advised me, my mates who are a bit older. There are many of us from my area, lots of people came here. (Daniil, gas-electrical welder, 19)

Alongside peer influence, place and locality played an important role in shaping the respondents' choices, as was indicated by the overwhelmingly localized nature of transitions into IVET colleges. Apart from a handful of respondents in rural colleges who had come from remote villages, the majority of the young people in the research had remained within their own district upon leaving school. To some extent, this was simply a reflection of the close proximity of IVET colleges to the areas in which the respondents lived. Since many of their parents had worked in major industrial enterprises, they had received apartments from their respective factories, and these tended to be close both to their place of employment and to their enterprise's college. As such, there were numerous cases in which respondents had made transitions into colleges that were attached to the enterprises where their parents worked, and in which they themselves would be offered a job upon graduation, with both college and enterprise being situated within minutes of their homes. While most of the respondents talked about such transitions in terms of convenience, however, their very localized character was also indicative of the close, symbiotic relationship between employment and place that characterized working-class lives in the Soviet Union (Clarke 1999, p. 16), as well as in Western countries under what Sennett (1998) calls the 'old capitalism'. Indeed, that the respondents' localities held for them what Raymond Williams referred to as a particular 'structure of feeling' was indicated by the common description of a local enterprise as 'ours' ('*nash*').

Echoing the importance of peer influence and place in shaping the respondents' college choices, choices of specific subjects were often rooted in informal knowledges shared by parents, siblings and friends who had previously studied in IVET colleges. In this way, while the social and cultural capital available to the respondents tended to localize their transitions, they were at the same time an important currency within the 'field' of vocational training. These informal knowledges were often co-opted by respondents into subjective hierarchies of trades based on factors such as earning potential and health risks:

> At that time everyone was praising this trade [machine worker], you know, 'It's good, it's good', whereas welder, everyone just warned me, 'You'll lose your eyesight', so I chose machine worker. (Ildus, machine worker, 19)

Of course, specific subject choices were to a large extent simply a matter of what was available. Depending on which college they were in, many of the young women in the study had only one 'female' subject to choose from, usually either sewing or cooking. At the same time, it was precisely the strongly gendered nature of training courses that allowed both young men and women to construct their transitions not only into IVET colleges, but also into specific trades, as a 'natural' process. This was most commonly expressed in the reasoning by female respondents that trades such as cooking and sewing would always 'come in handy' at home, a rationalization which served to reproduce the familiar 'double burden' of domestic and waged labour for working-class young women (Hollands 1990):

> A sewing machinist can both go to work and sew things for herself, you just need some material .... I don't buy anything now, I just sew things at home. (Maria, sewing machinist, 20)

Finally, parents played an important role in defining the respondents' options, both instrumentally and symbolically. The decision to quit school after the ninth grade, for example, had often been heavily influenced by parents who valued 'learning a trade' over 'sitting in school':

> **R:** Well, after the ninth class, my mother and father ...
> **I:** Did they help you decide?
> **R:** Well, yes. ... It's not that it was their decision, it was joint. After the ninth, we decided I'd go and study to be a metal worker, because there (at school), there's nothing to do, because I didn't do very well in the ninth class, so we thought, there's no point. (Dima, metal worker, 19)

This active role by parents in the constitution of transitions into the IVET system was accompanied more widely by a general sense of appropriateness and acceptability regarding vocational transitions that the respondents derived from their parents' careers and educational backgrounds. Indeed, the decision to make transitions into IVET colleges by the small number of respondents whose parents had higher education may similarly have been shaped by the fact that their parents were mostly employed in the base enterprises of their respective colleges, albeit as engineers and the like. This sense of appropriateness was most obviously apparent in the definition of choice-making through a notion of 'inheritance', with a number of the respondents describing themselves as 'following in the footsteps' ('*idti po stopam*') of their parents or grandparents:

> Well, my father's a welder too ... I knew that I wanted to do this when I was still at school, when the teachers asked what you wanted to be, I said I wanted to come here. This profession's just closer to me I suppose, because of my father. (Vlad, gas-electrical welder, 18)

> I just like sewing, my mother is a sewing machinist, my grandmother used to sew, and my aunt also trained in this college. I just always wanted to learn sewing. (Marina, sewing machinist, 17)

On one level, the ways in which the respondents articulated their transitions into IVET colleges were clearly coloured by a need to regain some sense of agency over processes in which many of them had had few real choices. In this context, a key resource in talking and thinking about their transitions appeared to be the ability to wrest a degree of control over objective structures, if only discursively, through the rhetorical construction of 'fate as choice' (Evans *et al.* 2001). While structural inequalities limited the respondents' options, however, like Willis' 'lads', nobody *made* them 'learn to labour'. Through the subjective inversion of 'hand' over 'head' work, expectations regarding future domestic roles, and relationships with peers, family and locality, the respondents actively appropriated the 'logic' of transitions into IVET colleges. Although constrained by the opportunities open to them, the way the respondents made choices within the field of secondary education effected what Bourdieu (1977, p. 72) terms 'the internalisation of externality, and the externalisation of internality', such that IVET students were like 'fish in water'. The transition into IVET colleges continued to be experienced as 'natural', an unproblematic socialization towards particular labour market positions and identities that closely resembled an 'apprenticeship' to an 'inheritance'.

Inheritance lost

> I worked [at the clothing factory] for a while but ... the wages were just awful, you had to wait two months to get paid, and then it was just so little, about 900 roubles ... we were just cheap labour (Irina, sewing machinist, 19)

> We haven't received anything at all for the last 3 months, we just sit there ... when there's work, we work, but if there's no work, we sit there, or they send us home for a month, maybe two. (Alsu, machine operator, 24)

> At the moment in our country you're not going to do anything without higher education – you're only going to work with a shovel in your hand. (Ruslan, interior decorator, 18)

Although the majority of the respondents described their transitions through IVET colleges in terms of affinity, choice and inheritance, the degradation of the opportunities at the end of the vocational track significantly undermined the possibility of realizing the labour market identities that emerged from this pathway. While they had experienced studying in the IVET sector as a series of 'confirmations', the prospect of working in positions corresponding to the level of their qualifications was for many of the respondents a 'contradiction'. Instead, the redundancy of the jobs available to them engendered a similarly individualized and diversified transition to that suggested by Cohen. In contrast to the commonality of experience in transitions through the IVET system, the respondents began to construct a variety of individual pathways and strategies through emerging opportunities in higher education and new forms of service sector employment, as well as migration to more prosperous towns and cities. As such, while these future transitions continued to be moulded by the same sets of resources and constraints that shaped earlier experiences, the 'normal biography' of a transition rooted in 'inheritance' gave way to one rooted in 'career'.

The shift from inheritance to individualization that takes place through young people's transitions from IVET colleges is best exemplified by the last quotation in the list above. First of all, the notion of manual labour as 'only working with a shovel in your hand' is reflective (although not indicative) of a wider attitudinal shift that has taken place in many post-socialist countries towards the near total denigration of working-class cultures and ways of life (Stenning 2005, Kideckel 2008). In contrast to, and indeed partly because of the ideological empowerment of workers during the socialist period (Lampland 2000, p. 213), discourses surrounding the post-socialist working class now bear a striking resemblance to the archetypal depictions of 'ghettoes of the workless and hopeless' (Reay and Lucey 2000, p. 411) that are constructed by the new Right around those living in post-industrial communities in the West (Stenning 2005, p. 984). In connection with this, post-socialist societies are beginning to see a palpable shift in attitudes to different types of work, with occupations associated with the old, 'heavy' modernity of the Soviet era sitting at the opposite end of the spectrum from more attractive forms of employment in the emergent service sector. In the present research, while established professions such as engineering had not lost their prestige, Western job titles such as 'manager' (*menedzher*) and 'merchandizer' (*merchandaizer*) carried enormous symbolic capital for most respondents, and left their own trades of machine worker (*stanochnik*), lathe operator (*tokar*) and sewing machinist (*shveya*) very much in the shade:

> I'm going to study finance (*finansy*) and credit (*kredit*) at university, maybe work in a bank ... I want to work somewhere where it's fashionable and where you can have a chat. In [our factory] it's like a closed box, you arrive, you work, you leave, it's like being locked up. (Andrei, metal worker, 18)

Alongside this shift, perhaps towards what Bauman (2005, p. 30) calls 'work as judged by aesthetics', the conviction that the best way of avoiding 'working with a shovel in your hand' would be through the acquisition of some form of higher education was widespread among the respondents. In this way, possible resolutions of the collapse of a 'collective' transition from school to work were located predominantly at the individual level of engagement with higher education. While old routes to adulthood had collapsed, the proliferation of new and easily accessible courses in Russia's tertiary education sector appeared to open up new opportunities for the construction of a variety of 'imagined futures', either as a route to new forms of employment in the service sector, such as those noted above, or to higher qualified professions in industry. That this was experienced as an 'individualization' of young people's biographies was most evident in the identity work that accompanied the respondents' pursuit of higher education, which revealed a more reflexive quality of identity construction than was apparent in narratives surrounding earlier transitions. Those pursuing service sector professions, for example, did not use the same life narratives when describing their future plans as those they had used to describe their pasts. While often identifying the rationale of the route that they had taken in terms of an affinity with manual skills, such respondents could rationalize present positions in a way that did not interfere with attempts at self reinvention:

> I need to get higher education, because then I want to go into management ... so it's really important for me to get higher ... but with sewing ... that's purely for myself, I just wanted to learn to sew. (Lena, sewing machinist, 18)

For others, and particularly those for whom the pursuit of further qualifications was unrealistic, there was not simply disinclination, but intrinsic difficulty in articulating their futures through the same logic they had used to explain their pasts, and a widespread questioning of this logic itself. While naturalizing the choices they had made through notions of affinity and inheritance, many respondents came to express major regrets about the pathway they had taken:

> I didn't want to study when I was at school, I just wanted to finish as soon as possible, finish the ninth year and go to college. That's how I felt ... I preferred it at college, it was better for me. Of course, now I think I should have stayed at school until the eleventh year .... But it's too late now. I understood late (*pozdno ponyal*) .... Now I think, I wish I were back studying at school ... I mean, what my life's like now and what it was then. It's like, I want to turn it all back. (Alexey, metal worker, 20)

In this way, despite the structural constraints on the pathways taken by the respondents, the contradiction between subjective constructions of identity and the objective opportunities to realize them was internalized as the product of 'bad choices' or personal faults. As Beck argues in relation to the individualization of life situations:

> Decisions in education, profession, job, place of residence ... no longer can be, they must be made. Even where the word 'decisions' is too grandiose, because neither consciousness nor alternatives are present, the individual will have to 'pay for' the consequences of decisions not taken. (Beck 1992, p. 135)

Indeed, it is in the individualized attribution of failure among respondents, noted in numerous other studies of 'working-class' or 'socially excluded' youth (Murad 2002, p. 43, Nilsen and Brannen 2002, p. 42, MacDonald and Marsh 2005, p. 196), that Beck's notion of social class as a 'zombie' category is most clear. While class continues to be present as a social division structuring the respondents' lives, it can no longer act as a social identity – as a resource and a narrative through which to make sense of and navigate not only one's past, but also one's present and future. In the new situation of 'ontological insecurity', class became more of a burden than a resource, as the respondents were required to 'plan' their way through new educational and labour market structures that required altogether different identities and forms of capital than those that had underpinned an 'apprenticeship to an inheritance'. As I explore elsewhere (Walker forthcoming), while the forms of capital available to the respondents were crucial in enabling them to 'get by' – in housing, the industrial labour market, and occasional prospects for migration – few were able to 'get on' in the ways that they had planned. Even those who were able to pursue higher education were ultimately more likely to experience the individualization of transitions from IVET colleges not as an opportunity to reinvent themselves, but as the source of new frustrations, anxieties, and 'self-produced' downward mobility. As Giddens (1991, pp. 53–54) argues, while the contemporary insecurities and contingencies that penetrate individual biographies compel us to retell the 'story of the self', we cannot tell any story we wish:

> **R:** After I finished, I entered [an institute] but I dropped out ... I studied for six months but didn't want to study any more.
> **I:** Why?
> **R:** I don't know. I enrolled for management. I suppose I just didn't want to do it.
> **I:** Maybe because you were working and studying at the same time?
> **R:** No. Sessions there are only twice a year, and the factory lets us go for those .... At first I was really keen to study, but then my desire just disappeared .... It's my own fault ...
> **I:** So you're not going to leave the factory, then?
> **R:** Not for the moment ... they've put me in a different section for a while, in cutting .... My friends at the factory say, 'Don't leave yet, wait – maybe they'll move you into cutting.' (Maria, sewing machinist, 20)

Conclusion

Bourdieu criticized Beck and Giddens for apparently extolling the advent of the 'risk society', arguing that in doing so they were 'instituting as societal norms those rules imposed on the dominated by the needs of the economy' (2003, p. 30). At the same time, he was also convinced that an epistemic (or 'epistemocratic') shift had already taken place towards a situation in which structural, systemic contradictions had come to find their resolution in individual biographies:

> Whereas the old system tended to produce clearly demarcated social identities which left little room for social fantasy but which were comfortable and reassuring, even in the unconditional renunciation which they demanded, the new system of structural instability in the representation of social identity and its legitimate aspirations tends to shift agents from the terrain of social crisis and critique to the terrain of personal critique and crisis. (Bourdieu 1984, p. 156)

This shift – towards individual self-censure and pathology in place of collectivist identities and modes of expression – is clearly evidenced by the young people whose experiences are described in this article. The aim here is not to romanticize the working lives that the apprenticeship to an inheritance led to in the past – a common criticism of those lamenting the 'end of work' (Strangleman 2007) – nor is it to assume that past social identities, however 'clearly demarcated', were entirely 'comfortable and reassuring'. Indeed, working-class youth were clearly attracted to the idea of social mobility during the Soviet period (Cherednichenko and Shubkin 1985), and young people in post-Soviet Ul'yanovsk actively welcomed the prospects apparently opening up to them in the new education and labour markets. However, while these emerging opportunity structures provided IVET students with a new 'language of choice' – one which quickly supplanted the language of class – planning one's way out of transitions to nowhere was no more likely than was social mobility in the context of the rigidly hierarchical Soviet society. Rather, the more meritocratic environment in which they now find themselves merely renders failure to realize those plans a matter of individual responsibility. As in Western Europe, the unravelling of working-class routes to adulthood in Russia brings about a form of reflexivity in which opportunities for self-reinvention are more spectral than real, and which only serves to strip away the language of class that had previously underpinned a sense of ontological security. In the post-Soviet example, in which institutional inertia and economic decline have rendered 'old' transitions simultaneously available and yet unviable, this disembedding of traditional identities and class-based narratives is thrown into stark relief by young people whose biographies are lived out between the old and the new modernities.

Acknowledgements

Many thanks to Hilary Pilkington for comments on an earlier draft, and to the guest editors and two anonymous reviewers for their suggestions.

References

Bauman, Z., 2005. *Work, consumerism and the new poor, Buckingham: Open University Press.*

Beck, U., 1992. *Risk society: towards a new modernity.* London: Sage.

Beck, U., 1994. The reinvention of politics: towards a theory of reflexive modernization. *In*: U. Beck, A. Giddens and S. Lash, eds. *Reflexive modernization: politics, tradition and aesthetics in the modern social order.* Cambridge: Polity Press, 1–55.

Beck, U. and Beck-Gernsheim, E., 2002. *Individualization: institutionalised individualism and its social and political consequences.* London: Sage.

Bourdieu, P., 1977. *Outline of a theory of practice.* Cambridge: Cambridge University Press.

Bourdieu, P., 1984. *Distinction.* London: Routledge.

Bourdieu, P., 2003. *Firing back: against the tyranny of the market*, vol. 2. L. Wacquant, trans. New York/London: New Press.

Cherednichenko, G.A. and Shubkin, V.N., 1985. *Molodezh' vstupaet v zhizn' (sotsiologicheskie issledovaniia problem vybora professii i trudoustroisvtva)* [Young people's first steps (sociological research on the problems of work placement and choosing a profession)]. Moscow: Mysl'.

Clarke, S., 1999. *The formation of a labour market in Russia.* Cheltenham: Edward Elgar.

Cohen, P., 1997. *Rethinking the youth question.* Basingstoke: Macmillan.

Coles, B., 1995. *Youth and social policy.* London: UCL Press.

Evans, K., Rudd, P., Behrens, M., Kaluza, J., and Wooley, C., 2001. Reconstructing fate as choice? Initial findings from the comparative study 'Taking Control?': personal agency and social structures in young adult transitions in England and the new Germany. *Young*, 9, 2–29.

Giddens, A., 1991. *Modernity and self-identity. Self and society in the late modern age.* Oxford: Polity Press.

Glendinning, A., Pak, O., and Popkov, Iu.V., 2004. Youth, community life and well-being in rural areas of Siberia. *Siberica*, 4 (1), 31–48.

Goodson, I.F. and Sikes, P., 2001. *Life history research in educational settings. Learning from lives.* Buckingham: Open University Press.

Goskomstat, 2005. *Regiony Rossii: informatsionno-statisticheskii sbornik, v dvukh tomakh* [Regions of Russia: statistical yearbook in two volumes]. Moscow, Goskomstat.

Kideckel, D., 2008. *Getting by in post-socialist Romania: labor, the body and working-class culture.* Bloomington. *In*: *Indiana University Press.*

Lampland, M., 2000. Afterword. *In*: D. Berdahl, M. Bunzl and M. Lampland, eds. *Altering states.* Ann Arbor, MI: University of Michigan Press, 209–218.

Lebedev, O., 2001. The Russian approach. *In*: European Training Foundation, ed. *Two perspectives on reforming the regional system of vocational education (based on the pilot project in the north-west regions of the Russian Federation).* Torino: European Training Foundation, 15–25.

MacDonald, R. and Marsh, J., 2005. *Disconnected youth?: growing up in Britain's poor neighbourhoods.* Basingstoke: Palgrave.
Matthews, M., 1982. *Education in the Soviet Union: policies and institutions since Stalin.* London: Allen & Unwin.
Murad, N., 2002. The shortest way out of work. *In*: P. Chamberlayne, M. Rustin and T. Wengraf, eds. *Biography and social exclusion in Europe.* Bristol: Policy Press, 97–114.
Nilsen, A. and Brannen, J., 2002. Theorizing the individual-structure dynamic. *In*: J. Brannen, S. Lewis, A. Nilsen and J. Smithson, eds. *Young Europeans, work and family.* London: Routledge, 30–47.
Reay, D. and Lucey, H., 2000. I don't really like it here but I don't want to be anywhere else': children in inner city council estates. *Antipode*, 32, 410–428.
Rose, R., 1998. Getting things done in an anti-modern society: social capital networks in Russia. *Social Capital Initiative Working Paper No. 6*. Washington, DC: World Bank.
Schwartz, G., 2003. Employment restructuring in Russian industrial enterprises: confronting a 'paradox'. *Work, employment and society*, 17 (1), 49–72.
Sennett, R., 1998. *The corrosion of character: the personal consequences of work in the new capitalism.* New York/London: W.W. Norton.
Strangleman, T., 2007. Nostalgia for permanence at work? The end of work and its commentators. *Sociological review*, 55 (1), 81–103.
Stenning, A., 2005. Where is the post-socialist working class? Working-class lives in the spaces of (post-)socialism. *Sociology*, 39 (5), 983–999.
Stenning, A., 2008. Livelihoods, assets and practices: diverse economies of post-socialism and the geographies of neo-liberalism. Paper presented at the Association of American Geographers Annual Conference, Boston, USA, 16 April 2008.
Thomson, R. and Holland, J., 2002. Imagined adulthood: resources, plans and contradictions. *Gender and education*, 14 (4), 337–350.
Tkach, O., 2003. The phenomenon of the 'Soviet hereditary worker': from asseveration of social class purity to workers' dynasty. *In*: T. Vihavainen, ed. *The Soviet Union – a popular state? Studies on popular opinion in the USSR.* Saint Petersburg: Evropeiskii Dom, 162–179.
Tomanovic, S. and Ignjatovic, S., 2006. The transition of young people in a transitional society: the case of Serbia. *Journal of youth studies*, 9 (3), 269–285.
Walker, C., 2006. Managing vocational education and the youth labour market in post-Soviet Russia. *International journal of human resource management*, 17 (8), 1426–1440.
Walker, C., forthcoming. Space, kinship networks and youth transition in provincial Russia: negotiating urban-rural and interregional migration. *Europe-Asia studies.*
Walkerdine, V., Lucey, H., and Melody, J., 2001. *Growing up girl: psycho-social explorations of gender and class.* London: Palgrave.
Wallace, C., 1995. Young people and families in Poland: changing times, changing dependencies. *Journal of European social policy*, 5 (2), 97–109.
Willis, P., 2003. *Learning to labour: why working-class kids get working-class jobs.* Aldershot: Ashgate.
Yaroshenko, S., Omel'chenko, E., Goncharova, N., and Issoupova, O., 2006. Gender differences in employment behaviour in Russia's new labour market. *In*: S. Ashwin, ed. *Adapting to Russia's new labour market: gender and employment behaviour.* Abingdon: Routledge.

Steps and stages: rethinking transitions in youth and place

Tom Hall[a], Amanda Coffey[a] and Brett Lashua[b]

[a]*School of Social Sciences, Cardiff University, Cardiff, UK;*
[b]*School of Music, Liverpool University, Liverpool, UK*

This article is concerned with the interplay of young people's biographies and transforming landscapes in south-east Wales. In particular the article focuses on a South Wales Valleys town, Ebbw Vale, to explore how changes to a place can be understood in relation to, and alongside youth transitions. The article reports on the ways in which narratives of the transformation, redevelopment and regeneration of place sit alongside the biographical transformations of young people themselves, as they make their transitions into adulthood. The article draws on concepts borrowed from geography, anthropology and architecture to advance a sociological argument for the consideration of continuity and everyday registers of meaning as a way of understanding change – both to place and in young people's lives. The focus on a place which has undergone significant material, economic and landscape change enables the argument to be developed in relation to the transformation of communities and post-industrial economies. The article thus explores some of the connectivities between young people, locality, and (both imagined and real) biographical and material changes.

Surveys of routes miss what was: the act itself of passing by.
Michel de Certeau, *The Practice of Everyday Life*

Introduction

The empirical basis to this article is provided by a research project which explored relationships between young people and the places in which they lived.[1] In particular the project focused on places undergoing economic transformation and, subsequently, community regeneration. The project worked with young residents living with and through material changes – to the local economy, geography, landscape, and social fabric – and generated a data set of ethnographic interviews and walking conversations undertaken in two primary research sites (the city of Cardiff and the South Wales Valleys borough of Blaenau Gwent). These data provided particular accounts of lived circumstance – personal, local and social – enabling us to locate young people's lives and biographies within, in relation to and in dialogue with 'their' place. Our aim in this article is to advance a broader, conceptual argument, removed somewhat from the specificity of individual responses. Our argument here has to do with the idea of change, specifically change as sudden disruption and discontinuity. Researching the impact of economic and landscape *change* associated with community restructuring and transformation, and working specifically with young respondents moving through a stage of the life course commonly figured as a time of rapid and significant *change(s)*, we have become critical of the idea of change as discontinuity or disruption. In what follows we make a case for the sociological importance of the recognition of *continuity*, as an underprivileged – often overlooked – and mundane register through which (young) people make and tell their (changing) lives, worlds and places.

We intend the article as a contribution to the sociology of youth transitions, and within that a contribution to sociological understandings of young people and/with/in place. The article also speaks to material, embodied and symbolic understandings of social class, as we focus our attention and argument on the South Wales Valleys borough of Blaenau Gwent, and specifically the town of Ebbw Vale. This is a place with a rich industrial heritage, a long history of manual work and strong community association; it is a place which embodies particular understandings and geographies of social class. The recent changes to the industrial bases in and around Ebbw Vale, and the associated plans for regeneration, raise questions in relation to employment, mobility and the rescripting of class and gender identities. In developing our argument in relation to the essentially sociological questions of change and transition – as experienced by young people growing up in changing and classed places, such as Ebbw Vale – we draw on extra-disciplinary contributions from the fields of human geography, anthropology and architecture. These perspectives enable us to work through some of the connectivities between young people, locality, and (both imagined and real) biographical and material changes.

The article is in four main sections. Firstly, we provide background and contextual material on our research locale, introducing some of the ways in which this setting (and thus our research focus) speaks to the connections between young people, locality, biography and class. In the second section, we draw on Thrift's (2005) work in geography to explore and critique the idea of 'step-change' as it might refer to changes in and of place and lives. In the third section, we turn our attention to movement and to the planning, mapping and plotting of change, drawing on Ingold's (2007) critical and anthropological exploration of 'lines'. In the final substantive section, we draw from the disciplines of architecture and town planning, in particular utilizing Cullen's (1961) concept of serial vision as a way of understanding changes in spaces and changes in lives.

The transformation of place

Ebbw Vale

Our argument in this article is more conceptual than empirical, and one which attends to the 'disruption' of change. However, it is borne out by ethnographic research engagement with young people in and of a particular place: South Wales, the borough of Blaenau Gwent, the town of Ebbw Vale. The South Wales Valleys, running in parallel from the Brecon Beacon mountain range to the coastal cities of Newport and Cardiff, constitute a geographically, economically and culturally distinct region, historically associated with intensive extractive industry and manufacture; 200 years of coal mining and iron and steel production. But not any more. Britain's economy has moved on – figuratively and literally – and left places like this in 'need' of 'regeneration' and reinvention in the face of economic and material change. It is fair to say that the South Wales Valleys have borne about as much of the brunt of post-industrial transformation as anywhere else in the UK over the last 30 years or more. Heavy industry is heritage in Blaenau Gwent today, if it is anything at all (see Dicks 2000). Ebbw Vale, the largest of the four big centres of population in the borough, provides a recent and particularly stark – visually stark – example. Ebbw Vale *was* a town organized around the production and processing of steel: *organized around* economically and socially, but also topographically. At the turn of this century, the steelworks – run down over a decade or more – closed for good and have since been physically demolished, leaving a levelled plateau at the centre of the town some 200 acres in size (Figure 1).

This has been a decisive and definitive transformation of economy and place. It is also a transformation to be (and which has been) responded to in policy terms. Economic, social and, in this case, topographical change, does not just happen, end of story; more often than not, it provokes, is responded to and acted upon. In the wake of change, Blaenau Gwent is now the focus of a welter of initiatives and interventions that can best be described as regeneration activity, foremost among which is the Ebbw Vale master plan. The Ebbw Vale master plan itself is a tremendously ambitious strategy document backed by the Wales Assembly Government, aimed at a comprehensive renewal of the entire economy and locality; a further transformation as seemingly breathtaking as any of those the town has already been through; a 'step-change' in the fortunes of the area, to use the language of the document.

> The Masterplan will create a new community in Ebbw Vale, vibrant with heritage and new opportunities. The redevelopment will create new places for learning, working and recreation. It will link into the existing fabric of the town and make strong connections to . . . important local landmarks. The site is being reclaimed . . . [and will be] replaced with high quality development and landscape. (source: Welsh Assembly Government website)[2]

Bold mission statement texts such as this often contain within them contradictions of the sort indicated in the quotation above – conjuring up a universality of ambition while seeking to incorporate opposed positions. In this case the contradiction, or tension, is germane to the theme of our article. Change – wholesale transformation – is in tension (or dialogue) with continuity. The Ebbw Vale master plan promises a

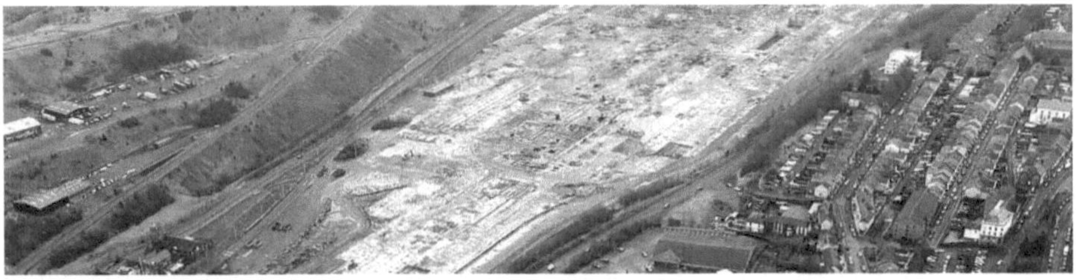

Figure 1. Former steelworks site, Ebbw Vale.
Source: Welsh Assembly Government website.[3]

new community in a place that already has one and an amalgamated vibrancy in which the new and the old, future opportunity and heritage, combine; the site of the steelworks is to be made over, but in ways which acknowledge the continuing landmarks of a familiar place and history. Here then are two ways of seeing change. As discontinuous, marking a break with what has gone before, and as continuous, taking forward that which already is. Of the two, the master plan is very much on the side of the former – step-change; it is pushing change (hence the concessions to continuity) in a context in which change – real change – has already happened.

Class, youth and place

Ebbw Vale, then, is a place, for our purposes *the* place, in which young people's lives and transitions to adulthoods are situated. Of course, we are reminded that in its exceptionalness as a place undergoing rapid transformation of sorts, Ebbw Vale also articulates to wider social and economic concerns with place and the geographies of social class. There has been a significant industrial transformation across many Organization for Economic Co-operation and Development (OECD) economies as employment has shifted away from the primary and secondary sectors. And accompanying this has been considerable social scientific interest in the processes and consequences of these shifts, including, for example, a focus on the following: the processes and policies of 'regeneration' (Hudson, Sadler and Townsend 1992, Beynon, Hudson and Sadler 1994); local responses to community transformation (Morgan, Rees, and Garmise 1999); and the ways in which workers, families and communities live through and engage with industrial restructuring (Fairbrother and Morgan 2001, Walkerdine, Fairbrother and Jiminez 2005). The fate of Ebbw Vale, its residents and community therefore belongs to a much wider narrative of industrial transformation and its consequences. There is no denying the dramatic transformation that this represents – from an industrial to post-industrial economic base, well documented through social science investigation. There is also a simple, if over-simplified, national economic and class geography within which Ebbw Vale is situated. To talk of massive industrial transformation in Britain is to talk disproportionately of north-east England (Beynon *et al.* 1994). say, or South Wales. Such localities were largely responsible for the making and remaking of the British industrial working class, and for the embeddedness and continuity of geographies of class and inequality. And in their post-industrial transformation, these geographies of class and disadvantage have not been done away with. Indeed, the economic and social difficulties faced by communities in the wake of post-industrial transformation can be acute. In this way, for many commentators, the task of understanding discontinuity – dramatic change and its consequences – has replaced an earlier focus on continuity. A sociology largely concerned with the 'problem' of continuity of inequality and class position – mapping these continuities and accounting for how they persisted as they did (social reproduction) – is now faced with exploring the fate of social class and social inequalities in the light of significant changes to (or the dissolution of) those very material and economic structures in which class identities have been formed and reproduced.

It is worth, at this juncture, returning to the 'place' of young people against this backdrop. It is well understood that industrial change brings with it particular problems for young people. For 30 years or more, successive UK governments have reacted to changes in economic fortunes and community transformations with a policy focus on young people – in relation, for example, to education and training, labour market opportunities, leisure and consumption, and family life and relations (Henderson *et al.* 2007, Kehily 2007). Moreover, regeneration policies and aspirations nearly always include calls to young people, in relation to the provision of education, training, leisure, and 'space'; but also more implicitly in relation to community sustainability and the real and perceived prospects of movement *away* from the neighbourhood. The sociology of youth transitions has also increasingly been faced with understanding (supposedly increasingly) fragmented social and class identities – whereby social reproduction has become a less than satisfactory frame for making sense of increasingly individualized trajectories. Young people's transitions to adulthood are increasingly framed in relation to individuals tracking back and forth across a number of thresholds (for example, education, training, work, family and consumption). Calls to individualization, reflexivity and biographical projects of the self (Giddens 1991, Beck 1992, Furlong and Cartmel 1997) have also shifted attention away from a tight focus on employment as the key to adulthood, towards a more holistic consideration of a range of public and private thresholds. However, in the face of these theoretical shifts in the experience and understanding of transitions to adulthood, we also know that for a small but significant number of young people, the possibilities of adult futures remain marked by chronic and continuing exclusion (MacDonald 1997). Young people's lives also remain positioned in relation to their place, their locality, and their neighbourhood. The Teesside youth studies of the last two decades, for example, provided rich illustration of the ways in which de-industrialization impacted upon the lives of young people, not in uniform ways, but almost always in ways which spoke to continuing narratives of disadvantage and social exclusion (Johnston *et al.* 2000, MacDonald and Marsh 2001, 2005). It is these concerns with change and continuity, in relation to young people and place, that we wish to explore in the remainder of this article, beginning with the very idea of 'step-change'. Before we do so, briefly, and so as to ground the discussion that follows, we provide an overview of the research data and methods from which we are working.

Pedestrian enquiries

As we have indicated, this article reports from an empirical research engagement with young lives and local regeneration; our research enquiries sought to capture and record the lived circumstances and experience of young people growing up with and amidst change. Although we have referred, above, to places (and by implication people) as 'undergoing' change, this is not an unproblematic formulation. The truth is that places and people do rather more than 'undergo' economic restructuring or regeneration: they live with and through such processes, engaging actively and purposively with them, questioning and countering where they can, while at the same time accomplishing a work of accommodation and reconciliation, winding the new into the known, into the everyday fabric of life – which, as we all know, goes on. This is a process in which change and continuity align and combine; and it is this process of (re)alignment that we have tried to document and understand, *in situ*. In doing so, our particular interest – prompted by the early and emergent character of the data, and developed as the research progressed – has been with the mundane registers through which change is experienced and accommodated. Accordingly, we have, for the most part, spent time and spoken with local young residents, seeking their views and experiences rather than those of the professionals leading and managing community regeneration and development schemes: everyday encounters rather than expert opinion (the distinction is stereotypic, admittedly, and sometimes blurred in practice). And, although we have cast a somewhat wider net, our principal research respondents have been local young people in their late teens and early twenties. Interviews conducted with this respondent group constitute our principal data set. A distinctive feature of the research has been the *pedestrian* character of these interviews – both literally and figuratively. The qualitative research interview is conventionally understood as a static occasion in which the conversation may range but those speaking stay put, preferably somewhere 'quiet' or out of the way (see Denscombe 1998; also Wengraf 2001). However, we have conducted most of our interviews out and about and on foot in the local spaces that our young respondents routinely move through. Although this mobile method has made for some practical difficulty at times, it has allowed the interviews to engage directly with the local (changing) landscape. Respondents have been invited to walk us around the sites and settings that make up their local landscape, talking us *through* the changes with which they are living and growing up. Elsewhere, we have described these walking interviews as three-way conversations involving interviewee, interviewer and also locality (see Hall *et al.* 2006).[4]

Our respondents have generally taken to the idea of walking interviews, not least because this approach has put the pace and direction of our enquiries significantly under their own control. But beyond this welcome disruption to the power differentials of research interviewing, we have, we feel, seen a further disruption. Talking on the go, moving through local spaces amidst all the mundane distractions and reassurances of place, has given our interviews an everyday and ordinary quality, both in content and character. The interviews have been a record of everyday talk – full of the usual hesitations, digressions and trivialities – about everyday matters; and although such matters have included, of course, the significant developments that are a part of what it is to be young and growing up in Ebbw Vale in the first decade of the twenty-first century, the point is that these, too, have been delivered in an everyday register: no more no less than part of the day-to-day experience of a life led in the continuing present. Given this, we turn now to the idea of step-change – decisive, sudden transformation – and ask whether this phrasing can be said to match the lived circumstances it looks to frame.

Step-change and critical moments

We take the term 'step-change' to refer to significant change occurring in a discontinuous (and often abrupt) way. The closure of the Ebbw Vale steel mill, and its associated economic and social consequences, have been widely understood in just this way, at least at the level of expert and public commentary. The steel mill is gone; finished. Over 200 years of history – the first Ebbw Vale ironworks dates to a business partnership established in 1789 – ended. Demolished; swept away. This is a language of rupture and of catastrophe. A step-change in fortunes is required because a step-change in fortunes has already happened. The Ebbw Vale master plan in this context is about starting over; it does not set out a salvage operation, but rather a new beginning – a step-change that will secure the future for young and future generations.

In a recent article, geographer Nigel Thrift (2005) takes on this notion of step-change, through a theoretical exploration of catastrophe – significant, sudden and discontinuous change (for the worse) – particularly as it figures in common pronouncements on urban futures. Thrift starts out from the idea that city life is precarious and that cities themselves, at least in a certain tradition of urban commentary (see Davis 2002), are always about to come unglued, and are always edging towards catastrophe. Against this representation of the city on the brink, set to take a fall, Thrift proposes a kind of urban robustness that resides in everyday practices. He draws particular attention to routine activities of upkeep and repair that, for all their seemingly triviality, constitute the very possibility of the city:

> various kinds of cleaning, all forms of building maintenance, the constant fight to keep the urban fabric – from pavements and roads to lighting and power – going, emergency call-out to all manner of situations, the repair of all manner of electrical goods, roadside and collision repair of cars, and so on. (Thrift 2005, p. 135)

These activities are a part of an unobtrusive infrastructure of kindness in the city; part of an urban everyday that escapes conscious attention even as it makes up a good portion of our everyday experience of the city. Thrift highlights this work of care and repair as a counter to the trope of urban catastrophe – the city in crisis, doomed, 'heading for a fall' (2005, p. 133). And if the activities he lists appear marginal and piecemeal – trifling, in the face of some of the grand, global risks which are said to menace the contemporary city – then here also lies their strength: they provide an improvisational response to the unforeseen, giving the city a flexible resilience 'when things do not play out exactly as it is intended that they should' (Thrift 2005, p. 137; see also Graham and Thrift 2007).

Thus, Thrift invites a shift in emphasis away from event and discontinuity and towards the work-a-day continuities of urban process. This brings into focus a side to urban life and the life of cities we might otherwise miss, not least because they are somehow less newsworthy. There is less of a story to things tripping along; and more of a story if things happen. Of course, Thrift's most general point can be applied to recent developments in Ebbw Vale (and similar settings) – and to the vocabularies and registers of catastrophe and step-change (to be found across political, academic and media output) that have accompanied these developments. At the very least, it can be noted that the closure of the steel mill, if final, was hardly unprecedented. And in fact the most recent, and decisive, closure was rather more of a process than an event. True, the mill once employed close to 15,000 in a town barely double that size; but the final closure laid off a much smaller workforce of 780 (and area unemployment figures for the period immediately following the closure show no significant spike). Today the site offers employment to 50 or so as the work of clearing, decontamination and reclamation continues in advance of the proposed new build. And so on. None of this is to downplay what has happened in Ebbw Vale, because something has happened, did happen, but life goes on and is lived in registers other than that of the dramatic and catastrophic. Thus, while we would want to recognize, and certainly not downplay, the very real impacts and consequences of major industrial and community change, we would want to point, too, to the particular registers of meaning that such sociological accounts often invoke and evoke – and indeed to contrast these with more ordinary and everyday registers. The process of change did not happen overnight, life does and has gone on, and often, at least in our experience of engagement with local young people, with little more than passing reference to the steelworks, the closure, and the plans for regeneration (hitherto largely unrealized). All of this is preparatory to our primary interest in this article.

A key analogy on which our article builds is that between the (dis)continuities of change in the life of places and those of change in the lives of people. Taking forward Thrift's redirection of attention from the dramatic to the work-a-day and ordinary, we can carry this shift in register across to young biographies, to the lives of young people growing up in a changing community such as Ebbw Vale. Here, too, of course, the language of rupture and trauma has a place. Thus, the authors of a recent study of Ebbw Vale and the impact of the steelworks closure conclude:

> The central importance of the idea of social trauma as provoking a long term crisis for the community cannot be over-emphasized. It is not so much a question of mourning as the effects of the closure on relating and how these are shattered by the closure, producing serious long term effects, relating to loss and fears of annihilation, passed onto the next generation. (Walkerdine *et al.* 2005, p. 2)

While we do not take issue with the very real impact of major changes in place on (young) people's lives, we do want to present a different discourse, drawing upon Thrift's rethinking of step-change and our own work with young people (the 'next generation' if you like, in the above quotation). Our research worked at understanding two sorts of change and the relationality between the two. Changing place(s) but also changing (young) lives; community transformation/regeneration *and* life course passage. And of the two, it is really the latter through which we have come to rethink the former. It is young people we have spent time with and talked to; our awareness and understanding of changing locality has been pursued principally through conversations with our young research respondents. We have not interrogated place directly, as it were. And what we have come to understand is this: that apparent moments of step-change, seeming ruptures in the life of places, often remain (for young people at least) embedded within *continuities* of community, association and place. The young people of Ebbw Vale are living with and through change, as much as they are stalled or traumatized. Our interviews with them are not a record of loss and fear. All our respondents, of course, knew and could talk about the works closure, although only a few felt themselves to have been directly affected; hardly any chose to take us to the works site itself, preferring to walk us around their own, very local routes and circuits. Some were indifferent, or even glad to see the works go; some recognized that 'a lot of memories went down' along with the demolition of the site (although not many of their *own* memories); indeed, some were more interested in the first 'green shoots' of regeneration – 'more shops and things like that'. Most were unclear about the details of the master plan and cautious about the likelihood of any comprehensive turnaround in fortunes: 'There'll probably be housing estates down there ... offices and things like that, but I don't think the biggest promises they've made are going to come through'; 'I think it's [Ebbw Vale] slowly going up. I don't think there's any, mass sort of oomph, but I think there's ... improving.' All these commentaries were interwoven with observations on and from the familiar and continuing terrain of local streets and spaces, and the interim schedules of daily life: home for tea, out tonight, college tomorrow morning.

The recognition of this tension between discontinuity and continuity in the understanding of community regeneration can be productive, we suggest, in relation to the general understanding of youth transitions. From the outset, ours has been a project about young people, conducted through relations *with* young people. Thus, change was always going to be on the agenda even if our research sites had not been chosen for that very reason. Wherever they live, whatever may be going on around them, young people are of an age conventionally understood as, in itself, a time of change(s); a moment of acceleration past life course landmarks. Well, possibly. And here is the analogy, where we see these tensions manifest themselves – and where sociological accounts of young people's lives are perhaps a little awkwardly placed. One the one hand, a sociology of youth (and childhood) has consistently criticized developmental narratives in which youth appears as a distinct life course stage separated out from adulthood and relegated to the narrative past (Henderson *et al.*, 2007). In this respect sociology could be said to set itself against discontinuity, insisting instead on the continuities of lived experience. Yet, it is in a way constitutive of the sociology of youth transitions, at least that it figures youth as a time of movement across series of steps and stages. Of course, the movement may be back and forth and the steps and stages may be provisional and messy. As we noted earlier in this article, the sociology of youth transitions has moved on from an earlier narrow focus on the transition to work as the principal, pivotal transition from youth to adulthood and for some years now has recognized a wider spectrum of interconnected transitions which young people must negotiate (see, for example, Morrow and Richards 1996). In doing so, it has even begun to undermine some of its own distinctiveness, arguing that transitions are not best apprehended as something particular to any one age and stage of the life course:

> It may be necessary to question whether 'adulthood' (or the statuses associated with adulthood such as domestic, housing and employment stability) are really final 'outcomes'. Rather they may be better regarded merely as the stepping stones of the 'young adult' that are as intermediate or transient as the statuses associated with youth.... The main adult outcomes specified by the youth transitions model (employment, partnership and independent housing) may themselves be transitory, intermediate steps only. (Coles 2000, pp. 10–12)

No final outcomes. But even so, a step is a step. To speak of steps and stages, however hesitant or intermediate, is still to employ a register that models change as a sequence of discontinuous events. Think, for example, of a dotted line. It seems to show a movement, but more accurately (and seen close up) it charts a sequence of incidents. The movement is not there in the line itself, because in fact there is no line, just a sequence of isolated occurrences which the viewer is invited to consider as connected and signalling movement. Again: continuity and discontinuity.

This broadening out of sociology of youth transitions, towards a wider interest in the life course, has linked it with sociological interest in biographies and their narration. A key distinction that sociologists have put to work here (Rosenthal 2004) is that between the lived and the told life, between the circumstances that an individual has lived through and the narrative sense that he or she chooses to make of these (see Chamberlayne *et al.* 2001). Tracking back and forth between these two can be a revealing exercise in sociological analysis. But again there is a tendency to discontinuity to the extent that such analysis tracks only between events – be they lived or told. Thus, the continued use of the critical moment as a tool of analysis through which to understand (young) lives lived and told:

> A wide range of commentators have drawn attention to the consequential character of particular events in individual biographies. Denzin (1989) talks about 'epiphanies' ... [o]thers talk of 'turning points' (Mandlebaum 1973) and 'breaks' (Humphrey 1993). Anthony Giddens employs the concept of the 'fateful moment' ... we use the term 'critical moments' to describe events in young people's lives that they or we the researchers considered to be highly consequential. (Henderson *et al.* 2007, p. 20)

Events, turning points, breaks, (critical) moments. This is biography as a dotted line, as step-change, sudden movements, a series of discontinuities. Talk of consequential events was not absent from our discussions with young people, but our respondents were also living in the mundane present, and only ever speaking from that moment and place, and, as such, were as focused on their *continuing* movement (through life, today) as on any point of orientation or destination. Walking with us from home, to college, to workplace – to sites of significance – they had things to say *along the way*. Mention of (dotted) lines brings us now to our second way of rethinking and complicating change.

Lines, plans and plots

Here we take a second extra-disciplinary foray, into anthropology and Ingold's (2007) historical, comparative and conceptual investigation into the life of lines. Ingold makes a key distinction between the moving, living line and static linearity. In doing so, he draws on the work of the artist Paul Klee; 'As Klee memorably put it, the line that develops freely, and in its own time, "goes out for a walk"' (2007, p. 73), whereas another sort of line hurries from one appointment to the next, 'every successive destination ... already fixed prior to starting out' (2007, p. 73). According to Klee, the latter line is 'the quintessence of the static'. For Ingold, such a line is divorced from the movement that produces living traces. 'It can exist only as a chain of connections between fixed points' (2007, p. 74). This is the dotted line we referred to above. A tool for plotting or symbolizing movement perhaps, as in navigation, but not a line *of* movement. Such a line is the 'epitome of modern bureaucracy, the dotted line ... [upon which] the movement of life is collapsed into a series of instants' (Ingold 2007, p. 94). This distinction between the fluid trace and the dotted line yields, for Ingold, a key distinction between 'wayfaring' and 'transport' as two modes of inhabiting the world:

> The wayfarer ... has no final destination, for wherever he is, and so long as life goes on, there is somewhere further he can go. For the transported traveller and his [*sic*] baggage, by contrast, every destination is a terminus, every port a point of re-entry into a world from which he has been temporarily exiled whilst in transit. (Ingold 2007, p. 77)

This is a development of Ingold's distinction between dwelling and building. For Ingold, life is to be found in continuity (in dwelling and wayfaring), not in steps, breaks, or dots.

Linearity, we can note, refers to the quality of consisting of lines. It need not refer to the quality of straightness of a given line, though the latter use seems to prevail, and certainly so in references to the nonlinear character of youth transitions. But what is so troubling about the 'nonlinear' line?

> The difference between drawing a line freehand and with a ruler precisely parallels that between wayfaring and transport.... In the first case, only when the traveller has arrived at a place can he truly be said to have found his way there. All along the trail he has had to attend to his path in relation to the ever-changing vistas and horizons as he proceeds. So too with your pen or pencil: you have all the while to keep an eye on where you are going and make adjustments accordingly. That is why some degree of twisting or bending is inevitable. In the second case, by contrast, the traveller has already plotted the route prior to setting out. To travel then, is simply to execute the plot. It is just the same when you draw a line with a ruler to connect two points. (Ingold 2007, pp. 161–162)

Is navigation, then, of joining the dots, really the best metaphor – it is certainly a popular one – to employ in an understanding of youth transitions; of the challenge that young people face in moving through a terrain of contemporary uncertainty?

At this point, we introduce a visual analogy, returning to our research site of Ebbw Vale, and the situatedness of young people's lives in relation to this place in and of transformation. Here (below, Figure 2) are the steelworks again (or to put it more accurately the site), as imagined by the authors of the Ebbw Vale master plan. The graphic plan sets out the way things will be when *the* transformation has happened, dividing the site up into blocks and swathes of shading to distinguish different anticipated land uses – for example, a learning campus, business and retail opportunities, residential areas, a hospital, public space and parkland.

As it happens (though it is really no coincidence), these land uses map rather well onto those aspects of transition with which sociologists of youth (and youth transitions) concern themselves: employment, education, domestic arrangements and residence, health and recreation. Land use as life course, biography even, as conventionally plotted. What we have here is a projected outcome, a destination. Not the processes and wayfaring of getting there. And when we do get the getting there, we get it as a schedule of separate developments and outcomes (as steps, stages, or 'dots'), as in the diagrams below (see Figure 3).

The close detail is unimportant here in relation to our general argument, which is just as well, as the image quality is poor; but what is clear at a glance is that change is

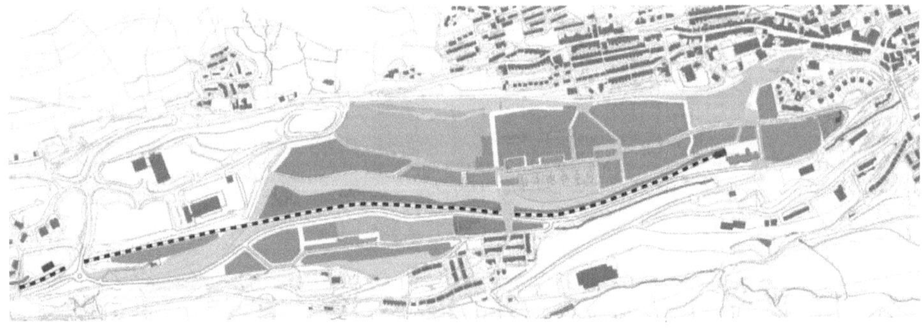

Figure 2. Steelworks site anticipated land use plan.
Source: Welsh Assembly Government website.[5]

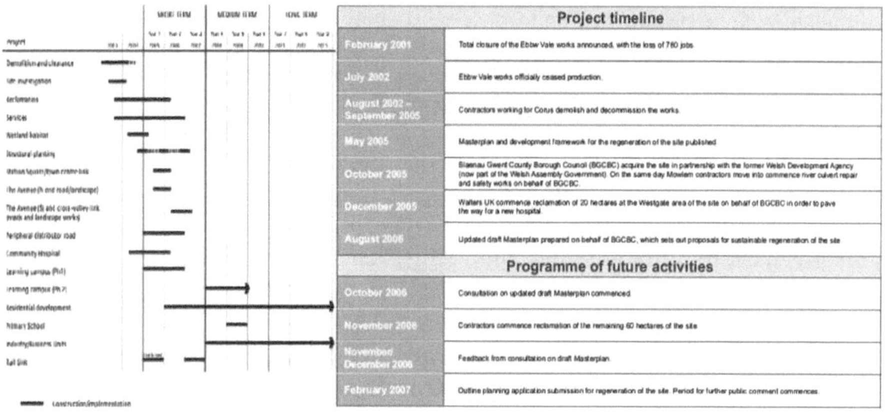

Figure 3. Draft schedules for Ebbw Vale master plan.
Source(s): *Valleys Voice* (community newspaper of Blaenau Gwent County Borough Council), Winter 2006; also Blaenau Gwent County Borough Council website.[6]

to be managed and delivered in stages, as a sequence of distinct activities. Straight lines predominate – guidelines, plot lines – and the lived moment, revealed by scanning the left-hand diagram from top to bottom at any given instant, shows itself as a (vertical) dotted line. Both diagrams purport to map movement, to chart change; yet they remain static, rigid, templates for change. Discontinuity prevails, not least because a well-established tradition of objectivity demands that this be so. Movement (change) must be apprehended – nailed down – and sequenced if it is to be understood. Such objective vision requires that the viewer get a 'fix' on the object viewed; thus, Ingold writes: '[i]n Western societies … movement is tantamount to "noise"' (2007, p. 136; see also Hall *et al.* 2008). And yet, it is this movement that characterized for us the ways in changes in place and lives were somewhat better mapped and described, as continuous flow, as dialogue, precisely as noise. To develop this further, we (re)turn to architecture and in particular to the idea of townscaping.

Stories, sequences and serial vision

In developing our thinking in relation to our argument here, we have found the concept of 'serial vision' (Cullen 1961) to be helpful. Serial vision is a technique that urban designers have conventionally used – for example in illustrated reports and plans – to demonstrate development proposals. Sketches of the way a space and place *might* look are arranged in sequence so that the reader can 'walk through' the possibilities. The architect and townscape consultant Gordon Cullen first coined the term and we have been particularly struck by the way in which it evokes space, movement and sequence.

> Let us suppose that we are walking through a town: here is a straight road off which is a courtyard, at the far side of which another street leads out and bends slightly before reaching a monument. Not very unusual. We take this path and our first view is that of the street. Upon turning into the courtyard the new view is revealed instantaneously at the point of turning, and this view remains with us whilst we walk across the courtyard. Leaving the courtyard we enter the further street. Again a new view is suddenly revealed

> although we are travelling at a uniform speed. Finally as the road bends the monument swings into view. The significance of all this is that although the pedestrian walks through the town at a uniform speed, the scenery of the town is often revealed in a series of jerks or revelations. This we call serial vision. (Cullen 1961, p. 9)

Serial vision is something like a story told in space. One thing (one view) happens, then another, then another; and it all leads somewhere, which is to say that serial vision has a plot or storyline. Of course, all stories are like this; they record in continuous narrative a sequence of unfolding events; episodes strung together along a line. It does not take much to see that lives and biographies have something of this same form and character. We tell our lives to others, if they ask us, as a sequence of things that happened: moved house, left school, went to college, bought a car, got a job, fell in love – a series of episodes. And again it does not take much to see that what is happening here is that continuous movement (through time, not space) is converted into a jerky sequence of events or happenings. This article, and the research that underpins it, are therefore (to an extent at least) concerned with a form of serial vision. The stories that we often 'tell' about lives, tend to skip over the bits between events where nothing much really goes on. But lives are lived in just these in-between spaces, getting on with life until the next thing 'happens'. And this is as true of (regenerating, changing, transforming) places as it is of (young) biographies and lives. For example, in thinking about the stories 'told' about regeneration – such and such a place was once like this, but then that happened, and then something else, and now this is planned, and the next thing to take place will be, and so on – we have episodic sequences of events. But, in fact, all places or localities, sites of regeneration or not, also have their everyday 'nothing doing' sort of existence. That is what places are like most of the time, and indeed are the primary ways in which they are experienced. To think it is any other way is to misunderstand what they are really like to live in. Our research project tried hard, in this context, to 'rescue' and record the life that goes on between events and happenings – in place *and* biography.

However, as we have indicated at various points in this article, we are also mindful that 'things' do also happen, and sometimes suddenly – to people and places; there is continuity *and* change, the everyday *and* the out of the ordinary. Thus, we have been interested in charting the sequences of 'events' in the lives of young people against the changes that have been a part of the planned regeneration of their local space. We have been interested to look at the ways in which these two do or do not fit together. Sometimes changes to lives and places have happened all at once and in concert; but more often there has been a mismatch of pace and sequence. This overlaying, in or out of sync, of personal and community change has real consequences and can pose particular challenges both for young people and for the aspirations and narratives of and for regeneration of place.

Concluding comments

In this article we have held back from a detailed exploration of young people's experience of place and change, as told through individual narratives. Rather we have instead sought to explore and interrogate the vocabulary and conceptual framing commonly employed in accounts of industrial transformation *and* youth transitions – in which discontinuity prevails, in which movement and change are represented as sequential. To talk of youth transitions as increasingly complicated, and perhaps out of sequence is not to leave the language of discontinuity behind; sequences and steps, critical moments and thresholds, whether these proceed in an orderly fashion or are shuffled and displaced by changes in opportunity and circumstance, remain as sequences and steps. Equally, to talk of industrial transformation as a sudden breaking off from what was and/or a step-change into a regenerated local future, is similarly to frame a local experience of change as discontinuity. And yet the research experience from which our arguments are drawn in this article has not been one in which our principal respondents, local young people coming of age in a transforming locality, have made it a priority to communicate their own lives, biographies *and* place as in any way disrupted by sudden change (to their town and their futures), or as experienced as a stepping from one key 'moment' or threshold to the next. This is not to say that the accounts of change that they have shared with us have been sanguine; instead, the registers they have employed have been rather more ordinary, neither blind to nor fixated on transformation. In calling into question the framing of change as discontinuity, we have not sought to set up a binary, in which one must side with either the continuities and ordinary registers of lived experience *or* the ruptures and jumps of change. Obviously (we hope), it is the relationship between these two that matters, and our contribution here has been to begin a recalibration of this relationship. Speaking from a research context of changing young lives in a transforming community, we have tried to insist on the ordinariness of change, as experienced by local young people. Thrift's appeal to local robustness and everyday practices of maintenance speaks directly to this recalibration of the dramatic and the ordinary – refocusing on the ways in which places and lives keep continuity in and through transition. Ingold's exploration of lines is also useful in developing this argument, both in relation to articulating the theoretical usefulness of non-linearity and acknowledging some of the discomfort of doing so. The concept of serial vision, of stories told and walked through space, provides a fitting – grounded, mobile and pedestrian – way in which to envisage the combination of sequence and continuity through which lives and places are experienced.

Our initial starting point for this article, and for the research which underpins it, has been to qualitatively explore the ways in which locality (place) and biography (young people's lives) connect to each other; and our substantive, geographical focus has been a place in which landscapes (economic, social, material, topographical) are changing – really changing in visible and documentable ways. However, through our research, and particularly in this article, we make a case for continuity.

Notes

1. This research was funded by the UK Economic and Social Research Council (ESRC), award reference RES-000-23-0878.
2. URL: http://wales.gov.uk/docrepos/40382/4038231141/1675529/1675595?lang=en [Accessed April 2009].
3. For a recent review of mobile methods, see Ricketts Hein *et al.* 2008.
4. URL: http://wales.gov.uk/docrepos/40382/4038231141/1675529/1675541?lang=en [Accessed April 2009].
5. URL: http://wales.gov.uk/docrepos/40382/4038231141/1675529/1675616?lang=en [Accessed April 2009].
6. URL: http://www.blaenau-gwent.gov.uk/theworks/masterplan/EV%20Ch%2009.pdf [Accessed April 2009].

References

Beck, U., 1992. *Risk society.* London: Sage.

Beynon, H., Hudson, R., and Sadler, D., 1994. *A place called Teesside.* Edinburgh: Edinburgh University Press.

Chamberlayne, P., Rustin, M., and Wengraf, T., 2001. *Biography and social exclusion in Europe: experiences and life-journeys.* Bristol: Policy Press.

Coles, B., 2000. *Joined up youth research, policy and practice.* Leicester: Youth Work Press.

Cullen, G., 1961. *The concise townscape.* London: Architectural Press.

Davis, M., 2002. *Dead cities: a natural history.* London: The New Press.

Denzin, N., 1989. *Interpretative biography.* London: Sage.

Dicks, B., 2000. *Heritage, place and community.* Cardiff: University of Wales Press.

Fairbrother, P. and Morgan, K., 2001. *Steel communities study: implications for employment, learning and regeneration.* Report to the National Assembly for Wales. Cardiff University.

Furlong, A. and Cartmel, F., 1997. *Young people and social change.* Buckingham: Open University Press.

Giddens, A., 1991. *Modernity and self-identity.* Cambridge: Polity.

Graham, S. and Thrift, N., 2007. Out of order: understanding repair and maintenance. *Theory, culture and society,* 24 (3), 1–25.

Hall, T., Lashua, B., and Coffey, A., 2006. Stories as sorties. *Qualitative researcher,* 3, 2–4.

Hall, T., Lashua, B., and Coffey, A., 2008. Sound and the everyday in qualitative research. *Qualitative inquiry,* 14 (6), 1019–1040.

Henderson, S., Holland, J., McGrellis, S., Sharpe, S., and Thomson, R., 2007. *Inventing adulthoods: a biographical approach to youth transitions.* London: Sage.

Hudson, R., Sadler, D., and Townsend, A., 1992. Employment change in steel closure areas during the 1980s: policy implications and lessons for Scotland. *Regional studies,* 26, 633–646.

Humphrey, R., 1993. Life stories and social careers. *Sociology,* 27 (1), 166–178.

Ingold, T., 2007. *Lines: a brief history.* London: Routledge.

Johnston, L., MacDonald, R., Mason, P., Ridley, L., and Webster, C., 2000. *Snakes and ladders: young people, transition and social exclusion.* Bristol: Policy Press.

Kehily, M.J.2007. *Understanding youth.* London: Open University/Sage.

MacDonald, R., ed., 1997. *Youth, the 'underclass' and social exclusion.* London: Routledge.

MacDonald, R. and Marsh, J., 2001. Disconnected youth. *Journal of youth studies,* 4 (4), 373–391.

MacDonald, R. and Marsh, J., 2005. *Disconnected youth.* Basingstoke: Palgrave.

Mandlebaum, D.G., 1973. The study of life history: Gandhi. *Current anthropology,* 14 (3), 177–193.

Morgan, K., Rees, G., and Garmise, S., 1999. Networking for economic development. *In:* G. Stoker, ed. *The new management of British local governance.* London: Macmillan.

Morrow, V. and Richards, M., 1996. *Transitions to adulthood: a family matter.* York: Joseph Rowntree Foundation.

Ricketts Hein, J., Evans, J., and Jones, P., 2008. Mobile methodologies: theory, technology and practice. *Geography compass,* 2, 1266–1285.

Rosenthal, G., 2004. Biographical research. *In:* C. Seale, G. Gobo, J.F. Gubrium and D. Silverman, eds. *Qualitative research practice.* London: Sage, 48–64.

Thrift, N., 2005. But malice aforethought: cities and the natural history of hatred. *Transactions of the Institute of British Geographers,* 30, 133–150.

Walkerdine, V., Fairbrother, P. and Jimenez, L., 2005. Regenerating identities: subjectivity in transition in a South Wales workforce. ESRC Identities and Social Action Programme, http://www.open.ac.uk/socialsciences/identities/findings/Walkerdine.pdf [Accessed 20 March 2009].

(Re)constituting the past, (re)branding the present and (re)imagining the future: women's spatial negotiation of gender and class

Yvette Taylor and Michelle Addison

School of Geography, Politics and Sociology, Newcastle University, Newcastle Upon Tyne, UK

The themes of mobility and transformation occupy centre stage in many sociological accounts, where 'movement' references people and places in 'new' times, often without situating how movements may actually be embedding or reconstituting inequalities, spatially, culturally and materially. Attention to how gender and class may be *re*configured queries straightforward notions of change, even 'crisis', pointing towards the reshaping of exclusions and their intersecting dimensions. Based on interviews in the North-East of England, this article aims to explore younger women's spatial negotiations in the context of change and continuation, where regional efforts on regeneration can be conceptualized against the backdrop of de-industrialization and (urban) rebranding; the 'past', 'present' and 'future' sit uneasily in these (re)imaginings. These reconstitutions force consideration of the different forms and consequences of social transformation, negotiated in the dis-identifications made by women where, for some, their presence was marked as distinctly out of place, as opposed to others who could more easily claim a movement and placement compatible with the sense of regional change and mobility.

Introduction

This ESRC-funded research seeks to explore women's lives in the North-East of England in the context of de-industrialization and the transition to a service sector, leisure-based economy. It investigates the emergence of 'new' femininities in a situation of industrial decline and regeneration, investigating what has so far been under-researched when compared with attention that has focused on boys' and men's experiences of these social processes (Wheelock 1994, McDowell 2000, Walkerdine *et al.* 2000, Delamont 2001, Nayak 2003). Industrialization has been supposed as good (for men) and de-industrialization bad (for men), and there has been little attention to women's positioning within economic regeneration/degeneration, the move towards and assumed fit into a 'feminized' labour force (Adkins 2002). Working-class masculinity, in the context of de-industrialization, receives increasing academic attention (Charlesworth 2000, Strangleman 2004) and features in popular culture (the film *Billy Elliot* (2000)), while femininity is positioned as a reserve, a labour market supply, which can now be capitalized upon, even as this has been named as a classed resource (Skeggs 1997). The themes of mobility, fluidity and transformation occupy centre stage in many accounts, where 'movement' references people, places and forms of capital (Bauman 2000) often without situating how such movements may be embedding or reconstituting class and gender inequalities, spatially, culturally and materially (Adkins 2002). Attention to how gender and class may be reconfigured in 'changing' times queries straightforward notions of (feminine) 'success' and 'fit' against (masculine) 'crisis', pointing instead towards the reshaping of exclusions and their intersecting social and cultural dimensions.

This article aims to explore younger women's spatial negotiations in the context of change and continuation, where regional efforts on regeneration can be conceptualized against the backdrop of de-industrialization and (urban) rebranding; the 'past' and 'future' sit uneasily in these (re)imaginings in both regional development discourses and interviewee accounts, as well as in the relegation of structural divisions (such as class) to the 'past'. It will be shown that such divisions persist and are actually reconstituted in and on the places occupied by young women, whether that be in exemplarily regenerated cultural sites in the main urban centre of Newcastle and Gateshead (such as the Quayside, the Millennium Bridge, the Sage Art Gallery, the Baltic Concert Hall) or in differently situated 'home' space. These reconstitutions force consideration of the different forms and consequences of social transformation, negotiated in the dis-identifications made by young women where, for some, their presence, appearance and selves were marked as distinctly out of place, as opposed to other, middle-class women, who could more easily claim a movement and placement compatible with the sense of regional change and mobility.

The persistence and discontinuity of class, spatialized, embodied and exemplified by people in (and out of) place has been explored, albeit often with insufficient attention to the gendering of such processes and (dis)investments. 'Displacement' has become a significant trope with regard to working-class masculine 'crisis', depicting, yet containing, all that is changing if not lost, in relation to forms of employment, community and belonging. Recently, for example, Nayak (2003) suggested that working-class boys in the North-East still 'perform' traditional, working-class masculinity, even in the absence of traditional jobs, subjectively making claims to a class-inflected 'Real Geordie' identity (Coll and Lancaster 1992). He traces how they negotiate the transition from heavy industry, as the main employer of the preceding male generation, to an unstable economic future that leaves their identity fractured, caught between the 'past' and the 'future': 'the 'Real Geordies' were like flies in amber, having become petrified in the hardened solution of an older period from which their values descended' (2003, p. 63).

For Nayak, this renegotiated, 'displaced' masculinity is evident in the growth of the service sector and the increased importance placed on regenerated, 'feminized' spaces of leisure and consumption. Football, he suggests, has almost come to represent the 'factory', with men flocking to the city stadium, enacting masculine displays as a reflection of 'Real Geordie' identity and solidarity. In their research on youth and urban nightlife in the North-East, Hollands and Chatterton (2001) also demonstrate the spatial production of working-class masculinity down 'the toon' in the notorious Newcastle city-centre Bigg Market site (which hosts various bars, clubs and eateries). The 'past', for these men, is both disappeared and re-enacted in the present, played out, even 'performed' on and against shifting landscapes and economic and cultural transformations. But a gap exists about how femininity is re-created in moments of 'loss' and 'gain' and how the story of change intersects with women's identifications and materialities. This question aims to ask more than simply whether or not women may also flock to – or away from – the city football stadium: the story of de-industrialization and increased opportunities for women also negates the differences between differently positioned women, leaving short understandings of how women are placed, and place themselves, within regional transition.

Savage *et al.* (2005) aim to understand the 'local' by exploring how people perceive residential locations, as related to different cultural fields, drawing from Bourdieu's notion of 'habitus', 'which insists that people's dispositions are embodied, and thereby necessarily territorially located' reproducing (dis)comfort and (un)entitlement in the person (p. 8). Spatial boundaries mediate locations and investments, giving people a sense of 'one's place', where in a mobile, global environment, location in fixed physical space may be of increasing relative significance in the generation of social distinction (p. 12). These competing conceptualizations, of change, fluidity and distinction, are of worth in considering women's own subjective 'sense of place', as well as the material realities as constraining and enabling these; this is particularly pertinent in exploring the place of young women, frequently held up as the 'can do' opposition against young men's 'failure', missing out the reinscription of class and gender division, beyond a simple binary of (dis)placement (McRobbie 2004, Nayak and Kehily 2008).

In unravelling how themes of risk, individualization and globalization are negotiated by young people in the construction of feminine and masculine identities, Nayak and Kehily (2008) explore 'new' forms of subjectivity embodied in changing femininities and masculinities. Young people are seen to use strategies of resisting, contesting and reinterpreting identities and spaces, in order to cope with restructuring and change: such responses intersect with many sites and modes of identity construction (race, religion, sexuality, work), often in highly uneven, complex and contradictory ways. In 'new times', Nayak and Kehily (2008) note the perceived increased levels of risk and insecurity posited by Giddens (1992) and Beck (1992) and the impact this has had on the construction of youth identities. They distance themselves from this line of thought, which claims that agency is set free from structural processes, marking the project of self-reflexive individualism (Adkins 2002, Skeggs 2003). While transformation appears to enhance the emergence of new femininities, appealing to subjects as agentic controllers of their own destiny, it frequently does so at the expense of those who cannot 'move' and are fixed as the failed 'Other' to a 'new girl order' (McRobbie 2004). Yet, Nayak and Kehily suggest that 'new femininities' *have* been positive and challenging to traditional notions of patriarchy, in contrast to masculinity in 'crisis'. However, using masculinities as a benchmark for the success of 'new' femininities gives cause for concern. And between femininities the marginalization of certain classed subjects can be witnessed, where local geographies, both physical and moral, contribute to the (re)construction of 'appropriate' femininity, spatially and temporally coded in the (gendered) 'past', 'present' and 'future'. Rather than detached, 'reflexive' mobile choices, it seems that classed and gendered geographies are embodied in individuals' sense of place, in feelings of belonging and in everyday identifications; they are materially enacted in the resources and opportunities that are available or denied (Southerton 2002, MacDonald and Marsh 2005).

It is these transformations which are explored in this article, drawing out what practices, resources and dispositions it takes to inhabit a 'cosmopolitan' identity, and what happens to those who are left out and left behind. As the spaces of the North-East of England transform, variations and inequalities persist in negotiating, resisting and even rejecting such changes; from accessing 'mainstreamed', rejuvenated, city-centre space, transformed by quayside developments, to happily living 'out in the sticks', women's own placements highlight the intersecting spatial, cultural and material facets of class and gender. It is clear that there are major disparities regarding levels of inclusion in the regeneration of the North-East – with some specifically excluded and/or simply forgotten. Thus, regional (re)imaginings, in terms of economic and cultural transformation, may negate the worth of remembered, ongoing identifications, foregrounding a 'mobility' that detaches its structural (im)possibilities, minimizing, too, the subjective 'structures' at play.

Methods: finding their voices?

Based upon 97 interviews (55 face-to-face interviews and 8 focus groups) with white working-class and middle-class women, this research overall explores women's varied (self)positioning within local transition/stagnation and the significance of gender and class in mediating identifications with 'past' and changing landscapes. It focuses on women's sense of regional 'regenerations' and 'degenerations', as classed and gendered accounts and experiences. Within the research sample, 66 women self-identified as working class, 22 as middle class, and 9 were reluctant to state or could not name their class position; the overwhelming ability to name class is, perhaps, testimony itself to its continued relevance, even as researchers report mismatches between subjective identifications and material 'realities' (Southerton 2001, Taylor 2007). Participants ranged in age from 16 to 85 years, a diversity aimed for, given that the concept of 'transition', so crucial to this project, is mostly explored in terms of (male) 'failed' youth transitions, effacing gendered legacies and changes between older and younger generations. In this article the thoughts and accounts of younger women (26 years and under, $n = 23$) will mostly be explored, but, in light of the focus on continuation and transformation, the accounts of older respondents will be briefly utilized: this is not to suggest a straightforward inheritance but rather to situate gendered shifts and legacies.[1]

Such diversity also allowed the continuation of classed experience and class (dis)identification across life courses to be revealed. The omission of working-class women from feminist analysis has been critically commented upon (Skeggs 1997, Taylor 2007), and is perhaps intensified in the academic focus upon complexity, change and 'risk', losing sight of 'old' certainties; categories become confounded and undone and that which was once foregrounded, disappears. This is true of class analysis, troubled and erased from the present, and sent back to the distant past (Bauman 1990, Giddens 1992, Beck 2000). However, the move away from fairly ungendered, quantifiable, socio-economic classifications has inspired increased attention to the cultural, embodied and spatial components of social class even as fault lines persist in conceptualizing the ways that social divisions interconnect, structurally and subjectively, as constraining and enabling (Taylor 2004, 2005). This is relevant here to the comparative positioning among and between working-class and middle-class women as they negotiate a changing economic and cultural landscape, with 'new' opportunities, spaces and identities available for some, as against the refusal, longing and unease experienced by others.

The North-East of England is an ideal location for such an exploration given its contestation, and enduring representation as 'working class' (Miles 2005) and the existence of competing public discourses on regeneration versus 'degeneration' in the North-East. For example, there has been recent debates on the relevance of the UK North/South divide as the North generates more wealth ('North–South divide "set to widen"', *The Guardian*, 13 August 2005; 'Renaissance for cities of the North', *The Guardian*, 31 December 2005; 'North just as prosperous as the South, survey finds', *The Guardian*, 8 December 2005). In such accounts, specific landmarks (such as the Millennium Bridge, the Angel of the North, the Baltic Concert Hall and the Sage Art Gallery) are often foregrounded, while others, both real and imagined, are dispelled and minimized. (City) space is regenerated and rebranded to feature on a global stage with 'culture' as a form of capital-building by way of a regional economic strategy, endorsed by One NorthEast[2] to improve 'international competitiveness'.

Rather than charting the 'move North' of affluence, culture and opportunity, this research seeks to paint a more complex picture of regional 'transformation' based on qualitative accounts of women living and working in the North-East. These accounts contest easy and sweeping claims to cultural ascendancy, as well as contrasting (and gendered) notions of the northern 'grimness'. Some parts of the North-East (both urban and rural) are still heavily coded as 'working class', and thus the interest is in the ways that women respond to, take up or 'lose out' in the resignification, resurgence and contradiction of and within the North-East.

The North-East has faced economic transformation in response to global change, impacting upon urban space, old manufacturing towns and mining villages; where the region was once built upon shipbuilding, coal mining and heavy engineering, it now relies on service, knowledge-based employment. The change in employment profiles – and the effects of this – can be aligned with spatial shifts, with centralized city spaces undergoing urban regeneration to accommodate new workplaces and workers, while other locales, both urban and rural, have lost out and are situated on the edge of such change (see Colls and Lancaster 1992, Nayak 2003 for a more thorough description and historicization of regional change). The focus was initially on three differently classed locales in the North-East (Jasmine Vale, Bridge Burn and Easter Hill), which were selected for their distinctiveness in terms of recent history, class character, and differing post-industrialization experiences. With these locations came a hoped-for contrast between a middle-class suburb (Jasmine Vale), a deprived estate (Bridge Burn) and a rural community (Easter Hill).[3] Over the course of the research, interviews were also conducted outside these three areas (including, for example, in County Durham and North Tyneside) – with classed differences, transitions and regenerations spoken of beyond and including those originally identified locales; classed differences were upheld rather than diffused in mapping spatial similarities and distinctions, with 'trendy areas' of leisure and consumption, frequently being positioned against 'no-go' city residential locations and 'backward' rural sites; claims were circulated and contested, becoming real in their respective misrepresentations as well as in their everyday occupation or avoidance.

We were able to approach a range of groups in these research areas, attend community events and advertise in general newsletters and newspapers all of which yielded responses. As 'locals' and residents of the North-East – and as researchers at an institution in the North-East – our intentions were rarely questioned. In using these spaces, the only criteria was often that we simply 'give something back': in working-class women's groups, this tended to be food and childcare costs (as requested) while in groups attracting middle-class women, we were asked to give more information regarding our 'studies' – and ourselves – suggestive of awkward and interesting processes in inhabiting differently classed local space. One residents' association, in the most affluent area, was particularly interested in academic credentials and abilities: 'how long had positions at the university been held and how did we come to be there?' Feeling ourselves to be classed in this way was revealing and dis-comforting; sometimes seen as comrades, as fellow professionals, or alternatively recognized as simply 'young'. There were palpable classed differences in the responses received, ranging from complete surprise that we could be interested in their lives (a much repeated 'why us?') to a sense that we *should* be attracted to and aware of their politically engaged activities.

The 'vulnerability' and over-researching of different groups was also differently demonstrated and negotiated across samples: one gatekeeper talked about women in poorer areas often feeling over-consulted by local government about area regeneration issues, and therefore being rather suspicious of institutions and researchers. The feeling of being monitored was very real for these women, indeed the numerous CCTV cameras on working-class estates were spoken of not as security but as a penalty focusing on their comings and goings – discussed especially in reference to benefit fraud. In contrast, another women's group, in a more affluent area, was well used to being consulted and listened to, having managed to successfully challenge the local authority on resident's parking and late-night drinking licences, and receiving media coverage as a result of their success. Differently again, the coordinators of one youth group (focus group 8) had such a hard time managing and responding to the everyday problems of their members that participating in the project was almost impossible and, at times, constituted an unnecessary infringement on their – materially and emotionally – constrained space and time. Such initial encounters served as a reminder of the efforts still needed in researching different women's lives, yet differences and inequalities were somewhat eclipsed in communicating research findings to local authorities and public sectors organizations in the North-East hoping to practise a more 'public sociology'; here expert audiences were convinced that the most pertinent gender issue was that of teenage pregnancy – a facet remarkably absent from both younger and older women's accounts, perhaps revealing the discordance between 'expert' and 'everyday' discourses and experiences. Here we suggest that comparative attention to the middle-class and working-class femininities being produced and resisted among women offers a way of theorizing the intersection of class and gender in women's lives in the context of de-industrialization and regeneration, resisting such gendered (mis)positionings, where the story is already assumed and/or 'written off'. It will be shown that gender and class divisions persist and are actually reconstituted in and on the places occupied by interviewees, whether that be in regenerated cultural sites or in differently situated 'home' space. The thoughts and accounts of younger women (26 years and under, $n = 23$) will mostly be explored in this article, with brief accounts of older respondents similarly highlighting gendered and classed shifts and legacies. This is relevant to a 'youth studies' approach, which aims to capture the influences upon and negotiations within young lives, in recognition of social, economic, cultural and spatial contestations across and between generations.

'The past is my present to your future': from the coal face to the car park?

Tired associations, continued (re)claimings

In the centre of Newcastle, set in brass in the pavement area in front of the monument to Earl Grey, is an inscription stating: 'The Past is my Present to your Future'. Around the edges, the words read 'Of Now, Of Then, Of Women, Of Men, Of Stone, Of Steel'; intending to reflect the connections (even disconnections) between these categories, we wanted to explore the relevance of 'past' associations and biographies in a landscape which is often automatically assumed to be male territory (Spence 1998) – where were the women 'of stone', 'of steel', were they still enduringly present or disappeared and relegated to the distant past? This landmark itself testifies to the connections between the 'past' and 'present', perhaps rewriting these on – even against – the transformed city centre space. But do shoppers notice this particular 'branding', as reimagining or 'reality', in the movement through central commercialized space? The juxtaposition – and suggested continuity – between the past, present and future represented on the urban pavement is embodied in Laura and Sheila's narration of space, place and belonging. Here, Laura and Sheila remember times and places now gone, recalled through their granddad's and uncle's 'stories'; for both young women, these stories serve to created a fixed sense of place where absent people and places are rewritten into the landscape, fostering a sense of belonging, a commitment to stay 'in place', to stay rurally 'out in the sticks'. Indeed, Laura refuses the promise of (urban) mobility, stating that she would 'never move to a city':

> **S:** I think the mining . . . there has been some kind of mining villages, so like all my granddad and uncles and things . . .
> **L:** Miners!
> **S:** So all the stories that I've heard, when I was little, is about the mining and the pit and even now, at the cricket club, where I go, one of the lads will say, 'Oh, I'm just a pit lad, me.' They make it out like it's a lower level or whatever but . . .
> **L:** I think it's nice.
> **S:** It's nice to have that kind of . . . that history.
> **L:** My granddad's from Easter Hill and he talked about, 'When we were lads, we used to go swimming here and that was all the quarry and they were the mines.' It's really nice to listen to it. I would never ever move to a city. Never. I like living out in the sticks. Right, there's nothing to do – it's what I like.
> (Sheila, middle class, 26; Laura, working class, 26)

Where the urban and rural have been separated in demarcating promising city space against that which is unchanging and 'backward', the declaration of worth and investment in the rural is notable, even as claims are specifically gendered ('pit lad'). In contrast to these young women's recollections and identifications with lasting legacies ('that history'), other interviewees spoke of the pit closures as an absence and a loss, spelling the 'end of civilization', where people were 'stuck' in place being unable to move away while awaiting for the return of what had now past. Diane's (working class, 51) sense of loss is narrated in terms of her husband's once secure employment, the passing of which goes beyond her own loss, affecting a communal decline: 'I think the closure of the pit really, spelt the end of civilization as we knew it.' It is difficult to conceptualize Diane's positioning through the logics of 'new' feminized inclusions, either economically or culturally; Diane's 'past' situation worked for Diane, even as its referencing at once foregrounds and undermines the place of the male breadwinner. This complex, and emotive, narration is suggestive of the significance of class, gender and generation in lamenting or celebrating 'new' and 'old' times, resonating with yet departing from Nayak's (2003) account of 'Real [male] Geordies'. Even those who inhabit this 'new' space, post-pit closure, still seemingly yearn for a return to better, past times, as captured in the above and in Ivy's sense of current misplacements 'It's like they're all still waiting for the pits to reopen even though the pits haven't been open in their lifetime' (Ivy, working class, 45). These accounts illustrate the pull of the 'past', yet there were various (dis)investments in enduring legacies, disputed also for their 'tired associations', where the past links were disputed rather than repeated, and rejected in favour of new, better relations. Charlotte (53, working class), for example, proudly declared that she was 'the one person who tried to stop *Billy Elliot* being filmed here'; rather than being seen as uncovering a neglected story, for Charlotte, this one had already been much repeated, to her irritation. Here the 'past' is put to rest in making claims to 'get on' and 'ahead', contrasting with the (younger) 'others' whom Ivy situates as nostalgically awaiting the return of a 'past' that they were never part of.

Cathy also rejects what may also be seen as 'tired' – though ever present– associations, written on to the landscape and onto certain (particularly women's) bodies. Her account disputes the sentiments of a shared past; this is devalued as are the 'new' spatial transformations exemplified by leisure sites, which are coded here, like the occupants, as excessive, rather than as tastefully cultural. Indeed, Cathy sees it as her 'job' to re-educate on past and present landscapes: it is this frustration of what was (not?) and what could be that Cathy seemingly struggles with in seeking to reimagine a more desirable landscape, resonating with and incorporating her own worth:

> I think people think we're all pit bulls and, erm, lower class, and that frustrates me. I make it sort of a job of mine to show that we're not all like that. And when you see, on the telly or anything, they're always showing like the Bigg Market, with people throwing up down the Bigg Market and things like that; I mean, that makes me cringe myself. I wouldn't go anywhere near the Bigg Market, d'ya know what I mean, so ... it annoys us that people show that side of the North-East and don't show that we're not all like that, we can do other things, we ... you know, we improve our lives, we do make sort of, erm ... there is some successful people amongst us that ... can move up the housing ladder and start their own businesses and do whatever – we're not all pit bulls and shipyard workers and things like that, so that annoys us. (Cathy, 47, middle class)

As Cathy's account demonstrates, the rejuvenation of the North-East via the consumption of leisure sharply highlights new segregations, with the 'wrong' people relegated and (mis)placed into the 'wrong' areas; gender and class are relevant in the reclamation and contestation of social space (Hollands 1995, Hollands and Chatterton 2001). For example, romanticized representations seeking to reaffirm traditional femininity ('Our Mam', Lawler 2000), exist alongside representations that problematize and pathologize women's sexual behaviour; their appearance in public, especially leisure, space; and their uptake of a 'laddish' drinking culture (McRobbie 2000, Griffin 2001, Harris 2004, Jackson and Tinkler 2005). These representations and discourses are relevant in the everyday negotiation of place where the landscape that Cathy rejects is one of classed and gendered excess, situated within the Bigg Market, often spoken of as a contrast to the 'right' places to be/seen (Quayside/Jasmine Vale), echoed in the adamant declaration, 'We're not all pit bulls and shipyard workers and things like that, so that annoys us'.

Place to be? Leisure economies, leisured selves

Rather differently, the young, working-class women in focus group 6 asked the researchers if they had been to the Bigg Market as *the* place to be, rejecting the disassociation made by Cathy, and actively claiming this as a place of leisure, where entry to this space would earn them a degree of respect and opportunity to meet young men. Sitting outside regenerated Quayside space, the Bigg Market is commonly represented as 'rough', even out of bounds (Hollands 1995, Chatterton and Hollands 2001), yet these young, working-class women found that this was one of the few places they could access and enjoy – even as this was fractured through gendered and sexualized claims and performances, enacted by young men. In the remaking of leisure space, and the multiple tensions reproduced in inhabiting (in)correct spaces, it seems that these young, working-class women have limited opportunities to reclaim sites; unlike Cathy, they lack the legitimacy, or cultural capital, to be able to authoritatively define and use such space. Their precarious positioning within the Bigg Market is demonstrated in the sexual harassment faced, resulting in a move away and a further containment of their leisure space. Such experiences problematize notions of a 'feminized' sphere, where men are adapting to new conditions and resituating their masculine identities accordingly; indeed, it may be asked how much transformation is really occurring when it appears that men are able to move, while young women in such spaces seemingly exist on the periphery, serving to confirm (or deny) masculine performances. Such young women are likely to be (mis)recognized as 'girls at risk', rather than successfully spatializing their 'new' femininities (Harris 2004):

Casey: We were in KFC [Kentucky Fried Chicken], right, and there were these fit lads, like, and they were absolutely drunk, right, this bloke right from the Bigg Market ... we were sitting in KFC, but one lad was proper fit, right, and he started agitating wor. Taking the mickey and that. We had a big bucket between we, and he called we all 'Fat Bastards'... And his friend came to the window and pulled his pants down – we didn't see...

Jo: I saw...

Casey: She saw – he put his arse at the window and he came in and he looked at us and he said as he started undoing his belt, 'Do you want to see my hose?' I said, 'No, you're all right.'

Jo: Aye we did like just run around the corner!
(focus group 6: Sophie, 16; Casey, 16; Jo, 16; Jenny, 16)

This feeling of surveillance, featuring more acutely in the accounts of young, working-class women, often created an uncomfortable atmosphere and a feeling that certain people just simply could not belong. Although some young women were conscious of danger and being moved on, residential streets were talked about as places they could 'hang out' and be themselves, 'You can sit on all the walls with your friends, all round here' (Jo). A feeling of anxiety, rather than entitlement, limited Sophie's leisure space: 'Don't really go out much, I just like ... if I go out, I go down like Jo's or Casey's or up Jenny's or something like that. I would never really leave the house unless I go to town or unless I go to the shop or something.' These narratives of uneasy and hesitant use of city centre leisure spaces were distinctly gendered and classed, contrasting with that articulated by more middle-class respondents, who could confidently name, and access, the right place 'to be'. This is evident when Jody speaks of the merging of – rather than distinctions between – spaces, where regeneration moves everything 'up market':

> So you see now this has, it's like the Bigg Market becomes Austin Road because there's all this activity and now they're making everything so up-market, you know, the property and everything. (Jody, 26, middle-class)

In this account, the transformative potential of 'up-market' developments are seen to spread outwards, encompassing 'everything' in their positive sweep. The 'past' landscape of the Quayside, what focus group 7 referred to as the 'smelly river Tyne', can be contrasted with the new, more respectable and sanitized development, contrasting Newcastle 'through the ages'. Many pointed to the changed Quayside as a 'revived and regenerated' space, with a picture-postcard backdrop, where the Millennium Bridge, the Baltic and the Sage were cited as impressive features:

> And I love walking down to the Quayside, there's so many sort of landmarks, literally all within however many metres ... I think it's really nice to take people down there, as well, like when they come up to the city, because I think it gives a really positive modern feel, like, it's quite like vibrant and nice places down there and things to do, so I like, I like that bit of it. (Gaby, 24, middle-class)

Gaby's uptake of space is connected to a sense of comfort ('nice', 'vibrant'), and an ability to literally 'show off', claiming ownership of and entitlement to such spaces and attractions: she views these sites, rather than feeling 'viewed' or surveilled by them as 'wrong', and unworthy of being there. Gaby speaks of these changes as 'putting [glamorous] new things on', to challenge negative 'grey', 'mining' preconceptions. Her account sharply brings into focus that which is reclaimed and put to future use, as opposed to that which is to be disclaimed and disavowed; such processes may be seen to be encoded in city spaces and indeed embodied in differently positioned women's uptake and refusal of certain places:

> And I think as well, the history, not just Newcastle but the North-East, everyone sort of thinks, 'Oh, it's grey, it's mining', you know, and it's not particularly like a nice glamorous place, like historically, but I think that's changing and when people come up, they're like, 'Oh God, this is actually really nice.' And you've not lost what it was, but it's like putting new things on it. (Gaby, 24, middle class)

While Gaby states that 'what it was' hasn't been lost, Jody (26, middle class) argues for a masking or removal of under layers, where such transformations would, hopefully, move the North-East 'out the doldrums'. Both these young, middle-class women, comfortably situate themselves in the 'present', with entitled orientations to future imaginings, rejecting the 'doldrums' of the 'past'.

Writing on iconic images of the Angel of the North, the Baltic, the Sage and the Millennium Bridge, which exemplify North-East regeneration (see Hollands and Chatterton 2001, Nayak 2003), the young women in focus group 6 commented on the 'beautiful', 'coolest bridge in the world', as viewers, while also feeling unwelcome as potential visitors ('never been'; 'rubbish art but good view'), yet this did not stop one young women from commenting on its 'ugliness' and 'posh slug' likeness (of the Sage Concert Hall). When asked about the Sage, the young women replied, 'It's just too posh for me,' becoming a space in which they didn't belong, 'I feel like an outsider. They're like, "Aaah!"'(Jenny). This feeling was endorsed both internally ('Because ... I don't like art. Just like "what the hell?"... But I've never been, I just think I'd feel like an outsider' (Jo)) and externally by staff and other visitors, who asked the young girls outright, 'What are you doing here?' Sophie goes on to explain their reactions to their feelings of exclusion, 'The Baltic? It's so tight, like if you do something like start laughing, then you get told off for it! And we're like "yeah? Do you have a problem?"' The following extract highlights their material and cultural exclusion, within such a space, where the young women prefer instead to use the lift and view the external rather than internal surroundings:

Jo: Everyone looks you up and down.
Casey: There's always old grannies in it and we don't like it so we just gan there to play in the lifts! ... And running round and taking the mick and dancing...
Sophie: It's dead expensive, as well.
Jenny: The café, like four quid for a drink...
Jo: We had fish and chips, me and my friend went for some chips, and the chips were like £2.20 for medium chips and the large were like £2.50. It's like, 'No....' It's three quid for a muffin.
Casey: I know.
Jo: You get your chocolate muffin and a cup of coffee and it comes to about £4.50 or something....
Michelle: Who are the kind of people that go there, do you think?
Jo: Old people.
Jenny: Tourists.
Casey: I hate tourists.
Jo: Lots of kids go there for... And you go in and you get these old women going 'Sshhh'. (focus group 6: Sophie, 16; Casey, 16; Jo, 16; Jenny, 16)

It is not simply the expense that is exclusionary, but also the literal and imagined silencing presence of others, whose gaze ('Everyone looks you up and down') the young women challenge, if not completely redirect; these young women may well 'hate' those who exclude, but this sentiment in itself is unable to affect the structural dynamics by which their own exclusion is reproduced. Such articulations cast light upon classed sentiments as a structuring feeling where 'categories of class operate not only as an organizing principle that enable access to and limitations on social movement and interaction but are also reproduced at the intimate level as a "structure of feeling" (c.f. Williams 1961, 1977) in which doubt, anxiety and fear inform the production of subjectivity' (Skeggs 1997, p. 6).

Residing inequalities

While such leisure spaces have been coded as exemplars of urban transformation (and indeed regeneration of the North-East more generally), signalling a potential and capability to become culturally, and economically advanced, such spatial transformation and rebranding also applies to residential areas. Yet where some places are deemed fit for inclusion in regeneration efforts, others are sidelined, existing on the periphery of transformation, where any changes may instead be negatively perceived by residents as 'degenerations'. In the focus groups conducted with young women, several identified preselected images of the North-East's past landscape as 'plain' and 'boring', while others stated their love of these same images, such as the shipyards revealing 'Newcastle's roots', identifying even with the 'depressing' streets, which were nonetheless 'sort of nice 'cuz looks like childhood', interestingly capturing the significance of a mediated past, which was not, given the respondents' ages, necessarily reflective of *their* childhood.

When asked to write descriptions beside other areas, beyond the Quayside, participants wrote words such as 'charver', 'rough', 'depressing' over Bridge Burn, while the descriptors 'posh' and 'student city' were scribbled against Jasmine Vale. The division between places emerged from interviewee accounts, as against wholesale 'improvements'. While Bridge Burn estate is architecturally famous, this representation sits uneasily with the gendered inhabitations of this as an everyday space – rather than abstract representation – where bags and purses may be more tightly held in passing through:

> I think Bridge Burn is somewhere where you're walking through it and it means that you've got a bit more of a sense of awareness about you, you know, you're a bit more careful, you might hold your bag a bit tighter; you know you'd be a bit ... like you wouldn't walk through it in the dark.... You see the Bridge Burn Wall is just kind of dominating your whole view, which I don't actually mind the Bridge Burn Wall, I think it's quite a landmark in Newcastle, but I wouldn't walk it at night.
> (Julie, 26, working class)

Jasmine Vale was often directly contrasted with Bridge Burn, mainly spoken of as a successful, vibrant, regenerated space, transformed from a middle-class residential suburb to a leisure space, with many restaurants, hotels and bars: however, distinctions between insiders/outsiders and ambivalences about the direction of the change in this area were also articulated. While resolutely identified as a 'good area', housing 'professionals', the commercialization of Jasmine Vale and the influx of students were seen to 'unbalance' the good mix of solid, sensible investments and (only occasional) drunkenness. The 'big explosion' in the number of students, was seen to change the 'ordinary' residential base of Jasmine Vale, and interviewees' spoke of being 'pushed out' and 'squeezed', emotionally if not actually. Interestingly, interviewees living here also spoke of the 'lack of space', of 'overcrowding' and of the danger of changing the landscape of 'building on a postage stamp' – worries that seemed in discord with where they lived and what they had, and such sentiments would perhaps be more expected from residents of, for example, Bridge Burn (given the physical overhaul of that landscape). Gaby and Jody also spoke of the manufacturing of space as false, where the place itself and the people within had to live up to the brand and were therefore suffering a 'branded' identity crisis. They situate the problem as one of outsiders coming into the area who lack the authenticity ('posh people who aren't from Newcastle') and thus entitlement to this space:

> **G:** Because they kind of built Jasmine Vale up, didn't they, and made it a really nice area but then put loads of students in. But it was like the posher side of the students, the ones you wouldn't normally expect to be at uni, like...
> **J:** Yeah, you know, like everybody with their collars up and their big pashminas on, strutting around the streets, and then they tried to make Jasmine Vale this kind of posh and upcoming place to go and drink with all these posh people, posh people

who aren't from Newcastle. Because when you go in Jasmine Vale, a lot of them are students from elsewhere ... the identity of it is not your typical Newcastle pubs, it's very...

G: False...

J: It is very manufactured to sort of be an image, it's like living up to the brand of Jasmine Vale, which is, like ... that doesn't sit particularly well with me.
(Jody, 26, middle class and Gaby, 24, middle class)

Jody and Gaby's account at first seems to contrast with the classed descriptors of places such as Bridge Burn and the Bigg Market; Jasmine Vale is under threat of becoming 'too posh' rather than 'rough'. Yet, it is this description, together with that of those embodying such an endangering aesthetic in 'strutting around', which highlights a similar grappling with classed claims and transformations in and on space, reactivating distinctions and exclusions.

Some spoke of the loss of the past, and were much more ambivalent about the changes in their immediate landscapes. Rather than articulating a notion of regeneration, women in more deprived localities spoke instead of decline and degeneration, where they had lost a sense of and claim to space, viewing changing locations as increasingly filled with the 'wrong' type of people; classed – and racialized – distinctions were invoked here to highlight who and what were still of worth in such (negatively) transformed spaces. Here, the young women in focus group 6 seem to reproduce a notion of entitlement and authenticity that they themselves were subject to, finding this to be exclusionary in their (dis)location from the Baltic Art Gallery. The numeration ('full of') and description of ethnicity and classed markers ('chaver') are suggestive of an excessive number of the 'wrong' bodies in space impacting on resources and a sense of (classed and racialized) entitlement. It is noteworthy that the comparisons invoked reproduce distinctions in the immediate working-class locale of Millfield, contrasted, too, with the middle-class location of Jasmine Vale, where residents are perhaps unlikely to negotiate such dynamics and discriminations, as alluded to in Sophie's comment, which suggests a distant onlooker removed from, yet gazing upon, such everyday tensions:

Sophie: In a way it's completely opposite because like in Millfield it's full of, like ... like, where I live now it's full of, like Pakis, like black people ... loads of Paki shops and everything. But like down Millfield and that, it's full of ... it's just like all white, full of charvers. When I lived in Millfield I only saw one black person in Millfield.

Jenny: I lived in West Dean for nearly four year and I was probably the only white person.

Sophie: I lived in Millfield nine year and I didn't see one black person.

...

Casey: I don't like my area.

Sophie: I don't think I belong in her area.

Michelle: Why?

Sophie: Just ... compared to my area.

Casey: Jenny doesn't like my area because it's full of Pakis. Jenny is a bit racist.

Jenny: I'm not racist.

Jo: She is racist, she hates Pakis.

Sophie: She thinks that they rule the country and have took over everything that belongs to us.

...

Jo: They get so many privileges though.

Jenny: Exactly!

Jo: If, like, the homeless and stuff like that. The council and stuff wouldn't help us get a house and that, but as soon as they come over from like Afghanistan, or something like that, they get a house like that!

Jenny: 'My village was bombed.' All they can say is, like, 'If I go back there, they will kill me.'

Sophie: And then they get a big house in Jasmine Vale, overlooking the whole of Newcastle.

While it would be difficult to dispute the racism within such accounts, it would also be simplistic to dismiss the narration of not/belonging and the differential and disputed entitlements which seem to intersect class and race, where a sense of the 'others' is spatially and materially mediated (Nayak 2003).[4] Lawler draws attention to the recent publicity surrounding 'chavers', which she claims to be 'a wide disparagement of the poor and the dispossessed' (2005, p. 800). The term 'charver' may be encrypted onto working-class youth, becoming synonymous with everything negative and uncontrollable in a community, where poor urban space is transformed into a warped fantasy of a 'no-go zone'. The young women also allude to the 'right' kind of whiteness, positioned against 'white charvers', yet this is an uneasy distinction as they may well be (mis)recognized through this, struggling educationally and economically and living on peripheral housing estates. In contrast, Angie's (25, working class) sentiments of what could easily have been ('they've had a hard life, and if you'd been in the same situation when you were growing up, maybe you would have ended up like they have, too') align her with her next-door ('charvas') neighbours, nonetheless causing upset in the everyday negotiation of home space, enforcing awareness of how demarcated 'no-go' zones – pitted against centralized, rejuvenated, cultural space – must necessarily be inhabited, negotiated and, often, filled with value. Angie's (mis)placement as she 'fights with' herself, points to uneasy negotiations which often reactivate and reconstitute inequalities and distinctions about who is properly in place, taking up or, alternatively, losing out in the resignification, resurgence and contradiction of and within the North-East.

Concluding thoughts: reconfigurations of class and gender in 'changing' times

Where the themes of mobility and transformation occupy centre stage in many sociological accounts, certain 'movements' are reconstituting class and gender inequalities, spatially, culturally and materially (Adkins 2002, Nayak 2003). This article aimed to explore the ways in which gender and class may be reconfigured in changing times, querying straightforward notions of 'change' and 'crisis' and instead exploring the reconfiguration of exclusions and their intersecting social and cultural dimensions. The dominant narrative of de-industrialization and the transition to a service-sector, leisure-based economy is one of masculine 'crisis', and necessary reorientation, against an often assumed feminized 'fit'; attention to how differently positioned women negotiate regional transformation queries this alignment. Much research on (youth) transitions has deployed the term 'transitions' to locate the structural processes of change located in educational and employment markets, lived out in the local landscape (MacDonald and Marsh 2005), where 'local' identities are produced in a 'globalized world' (Nayak 2003). Yet, 'youth studies' has experienced a separation between those emphasizing structural and cultural perspectives (MacDonald *et al.* 2001), failing to produce a broad conceptualization of 'transition' that includes intersecting social, economic and cultural processes: indeed, there is often an under-theorization of class and gender in such accounts of transition.

Regional efforts on regeneration can be conceptualized against the backdrop of de-industrialization and (urban) rebranding where the 'past', 'present' and 'future' sit uneasily in these (re)imaginings: places and people are differently rejuvenated, recuperated or rejected, included into or expelled from 'new' spaces. Such processes are classed, gendered and sexualized in that working-class women were frequently 'marked' as distinctly out of place, in both leisure space and in residential home spaces, which were typically represented as 'degenerated' spaces. Women negotiated such representations and everyday realities, evident in the distinctions and dis-identifications they made in making claims to (some) space. Middle-class women could more easily claim a movement and placement compatible with the sense of change and mobility; these are likely to be recognized as actively making use of space, investing in themselves and their landscape. Closer, critical attention to the inclusions and exclusions being reproduced here suggest reconfigurations of class and gender in 'changing' times.

Notes

1. This article focuses on a small part of the overall ESRC project 'From the Coal Face to the Car Park: Intersections of Class and Gender in the North East of England' (RES-000-22-2150).
2. One NorthEast is the Regional Development Agency.
3. All locales and interviewee names are pseudonyms.
4. Arguments about 'charvers' (or 'chavs') are complicated ones, which this article cannot do justice to here: others (Haylett 2000, Nayak, 2003, Hewitt 2005, Skeggs 2005) argue that particular spaces and places – housing estates, and places described as 'chav towns' – are used discursively as a way of fixing people in racialized class positions.

References

Adkins, L., 2002. *Revisions: gender and sexuality in late modernity.* Buckingham: Open University Press.

Bauman, Z., 1990. *Thinking sociologically.* Oxford: Blackwell.

Beck, U., 1992. *Risk society.* London: Sage.

Beck, U., 2000. *What is globalization?* Oxford: Blackwell.

Bourdieu, P., 1984. *Distinction: a social critique of the judgement of taste.* London: Routledge.

Charlesworth, S., 2000. *A phenomenology of working class experience.* Cambridge: Cambridge University Press.

Colls, R. and Lancaster, B., 1992. Geordies: *roots of regionalism.* Edinburgh: Edinburgh University Press.

Delamont, S., 2001. *Changing women, unchanged men? Sociological perspectives on gender in a post-industrial society.* Buckingham: Open University Press.

Giddens, A., 1992. *The transformation of intimacy: sexuality, love and eroticism in modern societies.* Cambridge: Polity.

Griffin, C., 2001. 'The young women are having a great time': representations of young women and feminism. *Feminism and psychology*, 11 (2), 181–185.

Harris, A., ed., 2004. *All about the girl: culture, power and identity.* New York: Routledge.

Hollands, R., 1995. *'Friday night, Saturday night': youth cultural identification in the post-industrial city.* Newcastle: Newcastle University.

Hollands, R. and Chatterton, P., 2001. *Changing our 'toon': youth, nightlife and urban change in Newcastle.* Newcastle: Newcastle University.

Jackson, C. and Tinkler, P., 2005. 'Ladettes' and modern girls: girls behaving badly? So what! Paper presented at the Gender and Education Conference, Cardiff University, March.
Lawler, S., 2000. *Mothering the self: mothers, daughters, subject.* London: Routledge.
Lawler, S., 2005. Introduction: class, culture and identity. *Sociology*, 39 (5), 797–806.
MacDonald, R. and Marsh, J., 2005. *Disconnected youth? Growing up in Britain's poor neighbourhoods.* Basingstoke: Palgrave Macmillan.
McDowell, L., 2000. Learning to serve? Employment aspirations and attitudes of young working-class men in an era of labour market restructuring. *Gender, place and culture*, 7 (4), 389–416.
McRobbie, A., 2004. Notes on postfeminism and popular culture: Bridget Jones and the new gender regime. *In*: A. Harris, ed. *All about the girl: culture, power and identity.* New York: Routledge, 3–14.
Miles, S., 2005. Understanding the cultural 'case': class, identity and the regeneration of Newcastle Gateshead. *Sociology*, 39 (5), 1019–1028.
Nayak, A., 2003. Last of the 'Real Geordies'? White masculinities and the subcultural responses to deindustrialisation. *Environment and planning D: society and space*, 21, 7–25.
Nayak, A. and Kehily, M.J., 2008. *Gender, youth and culture: young masculinities and femininities.* Basingstoke: Palgrave Macmillan.
Savage, M., Bagnall, B., and Londhurst, B., 2005. *Globalization and belonging.* London: Sage.
Skeggs, B., 1997. *Formations of class and gender.* London: Sage.
Skeggs, B., 2003. *Class, self, culture.* London: Routledge.
Southerton, D., 2002. Boundaries of 'us' and 'them': class, mobility and identification in a new town. *Sociology*, 36 (1), 171–193.
Spence, J., 1998. Women, wives and the campaign against pit closures in County Durham: understanding the Vane Tempest vigil. *Feminist review*, 60(Autumn), 33–60.
Strangleman, T., 2004. *Work identity at the end of the line? Privatisation and culture change in the UK rail industry.* Baisingstoke: Palgrave.
Taylor, Y., 2004. Negotiation and navigation: an exploration of the spaces/places of working-class lesbians. *Sociological research online*, 9 (1), 1–24 Available from: http://www.socres online.org.uk/9/1/taylor.html [Accessed 5 October 2008].
Taylor, Y., 2005. Classed in a classless climate. *Feminism and psychology*, 15 (4), 491–500.
Taylor, Y., 2007. *Working-class lesbian life: classed outsiders.* Basingstoke: Palgrave Macmillan, 2007.
Urry, J., 2002. Mobility and proximity. *Sociology*, 36 (2), 255–274.
Urry, J., 2003. *Global complexity.* Cambridge: Polity.
Walkerdine, V., Lucey, H., and Melody, J., 2001. *Growing up girl. Psychosocial explorations of gender and class.* Basingstoke: Palgrave.
Wheelock, J., 1994. Is Andy Capp dead? The enterprise culture and household responses to economic change. *In*: P. Garrahan and P. Stewart, eds. *Urban change and renewal: the paradox of place.* Aldershot: Avebury.

New class divisions in the new market economies: evidence from the careers of young adults in post-Soviet Armenia, Azerbaijan and Georgia

Ken Roberts[a] and Gary Pollock[b]

[a]*School of Sociology and Social Policy, University of Liverpool, UK;* [b]*Department of Sociology, Manchester Metropolitan University, Manchester, UK*

This paper presents evidence from the biographies of samples totaling 1,215 young adults in Armenia, Azerbaijan and Georgia, who all reached age 16 between 1986 and 1992, and whose subsequent life histories coincided with their countries' transitions from communism. The evidence is used to examine whether new classes are being created in the new market economies and, if so, where the new divisions lie. Economic classes are defined as aggregates with typical and distinctive labour market and work situations. The evidence points to the creation of two such groups, a middle class and a lower class. Corresponding social differences in family and leisure careers are identified. The paper points out that these emergent class formations are different from those in the West, and gives reasons why they are less likely to become politically efficacious than were classes in the West's more mature market economies during the twentieth century.

Introduction

What is class?

We need to begin with a stipulative definition. In this paper, 'class' refers to social inequalities with an economic base, that is, inequalities that are rooted in a society's systems for producing value and distributing scarce resources. These inequalities will divide a population into economic classes in so far as people tend to occupy the same positions over time; ideally, that is, in the extreme case, throughout their entire lifetimes. In sociology, 'occupation' is usually treated as the best single indicator of people's positions in these systems of production and distribution. Our occupations indicate what and how we produce, and simultaneously the rewards that we receive. Economic/occupational aggregates become *economic classes* if people occupy the same positions over time. If people were reassorted randomly between occupations each year, distinct classes of people would not be formed. Continuity over time is crucial.

Social classes (as opposed to purely economic classes) are formed when members of economic classes acquire distinctive social and cultural characteristics. There is never likely to be a perfect match between the economic and socio-cultural dimensions of class. Social mobility will usually result in an imperfect fit. However, if there was no connection whatsoever between the economic and socio-cultural dimensions of stratification, class would not necessarily be dead, for economic classes might still be present, but class would have ceased to explain most of what was attributed to class in twentieth-century sociology.

We shall demonstrate – we believe, without great difficulty – that classes are alive under post-communism. The main issues addressed in what follows are exactly which classes are being formed in the new market economies, whether these new classes share distinctive social and cultural as well as economic characteristics, and whether the emergent classes are likely to become politically efficacious.

Classes under post-communism

It is possible to place the populations of former communist countries within Western sociology's class schemes. People can supply the required information about their occupations, which can then be placed in the appropriate classes. A justification for this practice is that the same occupations have the same features that lead to their placement in classes in the West – relative rewards, autonomy at work, and authority over other workers (for example, see Evans and Mills 1999). However, the fact that Western-sourced class schemes can be applied does not mean that they necessarily offer the most authentic portrayals of class divisions in the new market economies.

Sociologists in former communist countries have agreed on just three points. First, most of the strata that were officially recognized in communist times no longer exist – nomenklatura and intelligentsia, for example. Second, the countries have acquired new upper classes, capitalist classes, usually locally known as the new rich, sometimes described as oligarchs on account of their control over politicians and political parties, and sometimes described as mafia on account of their ability to operate outside the law and their reliance on private security to protect their property and persons (see Eyal *et al.* 1998, Hoffman 2002). Third, they agree that the working classes have become politically, ideologically and culturally invisible – a stark change in countries which, until recent times, were officially workers' states, where workers' interests were supposed to be politically paramount (see Simonchuk 2004, Stenning 2005).

Thereafter nothing is agreed. One view is that after the collapse of communism the countries polarized into rich elites and impoverished masses (see Tilkidjiev 1996). Instead of using occupation-based class schemes, researchers have sometimes divided their samples into income quartiles or quintiles (for example, Bogomolova 1998). An alternative has been to ask people to rate their households' economic circumstances, usually in relation to what the respondents consider average, or to rate the extent to which they feel deprived (see, for example, Caucasus Research Resource Centre 2005). In Ukraine, answers to such questions show that during the early- and mid-1990s feelings of deprivation became more widespread and afterwards subsided (see Oksamytna and Khmelko 2004).

Other researchers have argued that entirely new classes are being formed. Piirainen (1998) argues that the main new schism is between households that now depend primarily on the market sectors for their incomes, and who consume in the private economies, and those who continue to depend on the state for their jobs or welfare and services. Khmelko (2002) claims that public officials who are able to use their jobs for private gain (sometimes by extracting bribes) constitute a new parasitic class. Kutsenko (2002) argues that experts (managers and professionals) with scarce skills and knowledge have become a new privileged class of workers. Ilyin (1998) counter-claims that the new 'holy' middle class is just a mirage, because when the new 'promised land' is reached, the salaries will rarely support a middle-class lifestyle.

All these claims are really hypotheses, backed by some supportive evidence, and they all identify economic classes without showing that they even possess the potential to become social classes.

Evidence

The data that follow are from a survey in 2007 in the capital cities and comparator regions in the three South Caucasus countries: Yerevan and Kotayk in Armenia, Baku and Aran-Mugan in Azerbaijan, and Tbilisi and Shida Kartli in Georgia. Strictly, all the results and conclusions apply only within the places from which the evidence was obtained, but our hypothesis is that the results and conclusions would be replicated in any other regions of the South Caucasus, and in many other places in other ex-communist countries. We have no fully comparable evidence from elsewhere, but such wider evidence that is available is always consistent with our conclusions about the main classes that are currently in formation, though, of course, there are variations by place, as we can illustrate within the South Caucasus, in the proportions of the populations in the different classes. We expected the main classes that were identified to be similar in all our South Caucasus research locations. This was on account of the similarities in the findings from all previous studies of young people in post-communist labour markets. If any of the locations proved distinctive, we expected these to be in Azerbaijan, especially Baku, partly on account of the historically Muslim culture in Azerbaijan (Armenia and Georgia are both Christian), but mainly because, since 1999, Azerbaijan has been exporting Caspian oil and gas, which produce revenue streams that have no counterparts in Georgia and Armenia.

The respondents in our survey were all aged 31–37 in 2007. They were all born between 1970 and 1976, and were members of the households that were studied in the 2005 Data Initiative Survey, which was based on representative samples from each of the places listed above (Caucasus Research Resource Centre 2005). The choice of age group to study was dictated by a requirement to gather evidence spanning the entire youth life stage, from individuals with little or no labour market experience prior to the end of communism. The respondents were, in fact, drawn from their countries' first post-communist cohorts of young adults. Our target was 200 interviews per region, and a total of 1,215 was achieved.

The fully structured interview schedule was based on instruments used initially in the British Household Panel Survey. The schedule was adapted for use in the South Caucasus, translated into the three national languages, and it was piloted and then amended. Fieldwork in all the regions was conducted by local teams of researchers. The interview schedule gathered comprehensive information from age 16 about each respondent's careers in education, the labour market, all paid jobs, marriages and cohabitations, divorces and separations, birth of children, housing moves and household composition, and participation in 13 specimen leisure activities. We needed longitudinal, biographical information in order to identify economic classes, since our definition of class includes continuity of experience in particular kinds of employment or labour market situations. We also needed contextual information about families, housing and leisure activities in order to explore whether any economic classes were becoming social classes. We collected no information in the quantitative survey that would enable us to explore the cultural dimensions of class formation, but we can establish whether the requisite economic and social conditions for such processes were emergent, and the following passages include some of the findings from 20 follow-up interviews in which the prompts included, 'Are there classes in Armenia/Azerbaijan/Georgia?' and 'Which class do you belong to?'

Analysis and findings

Career groups

We used two methods to investigate whether our samples had been divided into economic classes by continuous experience in definitive kinds of employment and labour market positions. The first method was based on time spent in different positions. Respondents were allocated to non-manual employment, other employment, self-employed, unemployed and inactive career groups according to whether at least 50 percent of their time since leaving full-time education was accounted for by these positions. Ninety-four percent fell into one or the other of these career groups, and the proportion of time spent in the definitive position was usually closer to 100 percent than 50 percent (see Table 1). In practice, this contained only 6 percent of the samples.

Our second way of dividing the samples into career groups was sequence analysis by the optimal matching technique. The best solution identified five sequences that closely resembled those identified by the time method – employed, self-employed, unemployed, inactive and mixed. Moreover, there was a very high level of agreement between the two methods on the career groups into which particular individuals were allocated. Both career typologies were good predictors of what respondents would be doing at the time of the survey. The results for the time method are in Tables 2 and 3.

Families, households and gender

During the 1980s, there was a fierce debate in British sociology over the conventional practice in class analysis of classifying entire households according to the male head of household's or the main earner's occupation (see Britten and Heath 1983, Goldthorpe 1983, Stanworth 1984, Abbott 1987, Leiulfsrud and Woodward 1987, Erikson and Goldthorpe 1988, Charles 1990). The case for classifying individuals rather than entire households, or taking account of all adults' occupations, had been

Table 1. Percentages of all time since leaving full-time education that was spent in each career group's definitive situation in the labour market.

	Non-manual	Other employment	Self-employment	Unemployed	Inactive
51–60	3	6	8	8	3
61–70	2	4	7	6	1
71–80	1	3	10	7	–
81–90	3	4	14	6	–
91–100	90	83	61	73	97
n =	290	101	166	391	118

Table 2. Career groups and types of current occupations (those with jobs at time of survey only) (in percentages).

	Non-manual	Other employment	Self-employment	Unemployment	Inactive	Other
Management	7	2	6	1	–	12
Professional	42	8	3	25	14	14
Clerical	47	13	3	17	7	20
Farm	–	4	47	3	14	10
Manual	2	67	23	42	54	30
Petty trading	1	6	18	12	11	14
n =	224	90	154	69	28	50

strengthened by rising rates of female employment, and more people living singly due to later ages of marriage and higher rates of divorce and separation, thereby making males' and females' resources and security dependent on their own qualifications, occupations and earnings. Since the 1980s, most sociological researchers in Britain and other Western countries have opted for individual classification.

The case for abandoning sociology's pre-1980s conventional practice is far less persuasive in the South Caucasus (and probably in most other ex-communist countries), even though under the old system around half the workforces were female. Formally, males and females had equal access to all programmes in education and occupations, but, in practice, there was considerable segmentation by gender, and women tended to employed in lower-paid occupations. All this has continued to be the case under post-communism (see Predborska 2005, Trapido 2007). In our research, the women who were in employment at the time of the fieldwork tended to be earning less than the men (see Table 4). This applied overall and within each of the three occupational groups, where there were sufficient numbers of both sexes (who also supplied details about their incomes) to permit meaningful comparisons.

The income figures in Table 4, and elsewhere when income is reported, are based on information supplied by our respondents. They were asked to select from show cards the bands into which their monthly incomes fell under a set of headings (main jobs, other jobs, grants, benefits, parents, etc.). The reported figures, as expected, were clearly underestimates. Respondents may have given their official rather than

Table 3. Career groups and current labour market status (in percentages).

	Non-manual	Other employment	Self-employment	Unemployment	Inactive	Other
Full-time job	68	55	8	10	4	27
Part-time job	8	7	3	2	2	3
Self-employed	4	10	82	4	–	31
Unemployed	5	13	4	62	2	11
Other	15	15	3	22	92	28
n =	271	123	163	384	118	62

Table 4. Occupations and (adjusted) total reported personal incomes per month at time of survey, in $US (in percentages).

a. Males

	Management	Professional	Other non-manual	Manual	Farm work	Petty trading
Up to 300	12	28	16	22	77	26
301–500	40	51	55	61	17	47
Over 500	48	21	29	17	7	26
n =	25	47	55	106	30	34
a. Females						
Up to 300		48	37	48		
301–500		44	46	48		
Over 500		8	17	4		
n =	5	71	70	25	9	10

their actual earnings (there is usually a difference in all the new market economies). We also enquired about their entire households' total monthly incomes and expenditures (again using show cards and sets of income/spending bands). Reported household expenditure usually exceeds reported income by between two and four times. This ratio has been used to adjust each respondent's personal reported income. We consider these figures unreliable at an individual level, but the resultant range of incomes looks realistic (consistent with other economic data from the countries), and the differences between socio-demographic groups are the same as if we had used the raw reported data. These differences, in our view, represent the real situation.

Since the end of communism, female rates of employment appear to have declined in all the countries, and women's rates of unemployment and inactivity have risen. This has not been due to women celebrating their new freedom to live 'normally' as housewives. Rather, it has been due to the loss of free or heavily subsidized nurseries and kindergartens, and private sector employers' reluctance to finance maternity leave and to treat female employees indulgently out of respect for their domestic responsibilities (see Bridger *et al.* 1996). At the time of our fieldwork, the women were far less likely than the men to be in employment (see Table 5). The women were more likely than the men to be in both the unemployed and inactive labour market groups.

Table 5. Labour market status at time of survey (in percentages).

	Males, capitals	Females, capitals	Males, regions	Females, regions
Employed	55	39	25	17
Self-employed	20	4	33	14
Unemployed	12	20	28	38
Inactive	3	36	4	28
Other	10	1	11	3
n =	225	320	269	307

In each of the research regions, women were more likely than men to be employed in the public sectors (see Table 6), especially in public sector professions, in education, health care, etc. The public sectors were where women were most likely to be able to take maternity leave without jeopardizing their employment careers, and to expect traditional (as under communism) indulgent treatment by their employers. However, males' overall greater likelihood of being in employment and their higher earnings, meant that males were normally their households' main providers.

It is also relevant here that most of our respondents had continued to live with their parents (or parents-in-law) until they were beyond age 30 (see Roberts *et al.* 2009a). This was most common in Armenia and Georgia (80 percent in Yerevan, 78 percent in Kotayk, 81 percent in Tbilisi and 84 percent in Shida Kartli), but even in Azerbaijan it was the statistical norm in both research regions (55 percent in Baku and 72 percent in Aran-Mugan). Majorities were still living with parents regardless of whether they were single, a couple, or a couple with children. Multi-generation living may have been a traditional and continuing cultural preference in the South Caucasus, but it had been normal everywhere under communism due to housing shortages, and subsequently it has remained common due to most young singles and even couples being unable to afford to buy or even to rent independent accommodation. There are some advantages for all concerned in multi-generation living. Household costs can be pooled (as can incomes). Assistance is available with childcare. Previous research has shown that the multi-generation household tends to transmit traditional gender roles and divisions down the generations (Tomanovic and Ignjatovic 2006). It most likely also helps to maintain conventional patterns of family life stage transitions. Across our combined samples, only 9 percent (though more in Georgia – 18 percent in Tbilisi and 12 percent in Shida Kartli), had departed from the conventional sequence from being single to becoming a couple (just once), and then having children and remaining a couple.

This means that decisions such as whether to marry and whom to marry were being made by individuals in family households rather than solitary individuals and couples (see also Wallace 2002). This also applied to decisions to attend university. This would usually involve family support – paying fees, providing spending money,

Table 6. Currently employed respondents: sectors of employment (in percentages).

a. Males

	Yerevan	Kotayk	Baku	Aran-Mugan	Tbilisi	Shida Kartli
Private	72	72	55	76	71	90
Public	28	28	45	24	22	10
NGOs	–	–	–	–	8	–
n –	64	47	55	45	51	64

b. Females

	Yerevan	Kotayk	Baku	Aran-Mugan	Tbilisi	Shida Kartli
Private	52	59	27	21	48	70
Public	48	41	73	79	50	28
NGOs	–	–	–	–	2	2
n =	58	37	22	14	54	43

NGO: non-governmental organization.

continuing to feed and clothe the student, etc. The likelihood of our respondents having progressed through higher education depended greatly on the status of their families. We constructed a family socio-economic status (SES) scale by awarding up to four points depending on whether respondents' mothers and fathers were higher education graduates, and whether their normal occupations had been or still were management or professional. This scale was then collapsed into lower, intermediate and higher SES groups, from which 21, 40 and 69 percent, respectively, among the young people had progressed through higher education to at least BA level. Investing in higher education was usually investing in a person who would remain a family household member, quite likely indefinitely in the case of males, and females also if they remained unmarried. Young people themselves, of course, could decide, but in the context of families where the parents had particular expectations and aspirations, and from which different levels of support would be forthcoming. Irrespective of family SES, higher education had increased the likelihood of our respondents entering the non-manual career group. Independently of whether they had progressed through higher education, family SES (low or high) also diminished or increased this likelihood (Table 7).

The new middle class

The young women were far more likely than the young men to have become university graduates except in Azerbaijan, the traditionally Muslim country in our study, and also where higher education was under much tighter state regulation than in Armenia and Georgia (see Table 8). In both Azerbaijan regions, roughly equal proportions of males and females were university graduates, and in both sexes far fewer than their Armenia and Georgia counterparts. The latter countries had experienced unregulated expansion of higher education during the 1990s, and the proportions of females attending university had risen well above male levels. These South Caucasus countries can be regarded as extreme cases of a trend towards females out-performing males in education that has occurred in many parts of the world. Our extreme cases offer a plausible explanation. Unless they had attended university, young women were unlikely to gain any stable employment, whereas with university qualifications they could enter public-sector professions and other non-manual, public-sector occupations, which, as explained earlier, have held special attractions for women (see Table 9). Azerbaijan, with far fewer female university graduates, had far more inactive and unemployed females in their 20s and 30s. Needless to say, as elsewhere, higher education was also a 'marriage market' (see Blossfeld and Timm 2003).

This meant that in the South Caucasus an archetypal middle-class household contained male and female graduates, very likely both doing non-manual jobs, especially the women, with males being more likely to work in the private sector or to be self-employed. We suggest that while necessarily collecting evidence from individuals, and while occupations may be the best single indicators of class positions, occupation does not equal class. Classes, economic classes in the first instance, are formed through the interrelationships between different inequalities including the occupations and earnings of different household members, and social classes are formed through sharing other common experiences such as middle-class family backgrounds and childhoods, and higher education. Classes contain relatively solid cores, and there are peripheries where household class connections are weaker

Table 7. Parental class, education and labour market careers (in percentages).

	Low class, higher education	Low class, other	Intermediate class, higher education	Intermediate class, other	High class, higher education	High class, other
Non-manual employment	28	8	45	23	54	32
Other employment	13	13	9	12	10	6
Self-employment	8	21	3	17	5	19
Unemployment	44	39	29	30	20	27
Non-active	6	14	8	9	7	10
Other	3	6	6	9	4	6
n =	119	447	161	235	140	63

Table 8. Percentages of males and females with higher education by region.

	Males	Females
Armenia		
Yerevan	35%	58%
Kotayk	29%	50%
Azerbaijan		
Baku	28%	27%
Aran-Mugan	11%	10%
Georgia		
Tbilisi	49%	62%
Shida Kartli	26%	34%

and often ambiguous. One such core that can be identified in our research in the South Caucasus is a middle-class core. According to our evidence, the new 'holy' middle class is not a mirage.

If the family household is treated as the classed unit, we recognize the implausibility of specific sections of the non-manual workforces developing into distinct classes: expert professionals and managers, bribe-taking public officials, or a class break between private and public sector employees. It is unlikely that only one type of middle-class employment will be represented within a middle-class family household. The case for not separating professionals and managers (a service class) from other non-manuals also becomes clear. In the South Caucasus it was rare for anyone who was not acting directly in the place of the owner of an enterprise to be described as a manager, so there were few of them: 14 percent of male employees in the capitals but only 3 percent of the females, and just 2 percent of male employees in the non-capital regions and no females whatsoever. 'Professional', in these countries, meant working according to one's specialty (acquired in higher education), which was nearly always in the public sector, and these jobs were generally lower paid than other non-manual occupations: the professional positions tended to be occupied by women. Non-manual employment in general was the only plausible base for an economic middle class. We will consider shortly whether this middle class had acquired any further characteristics of a social class.

Table 9. Occupations of respondents in jobs at time of survey (in percentages).

	Males, capitals	Females, capitals	Males, regions	Females, regions
Management	14	3	2	–
Professional	12	33	15	37
Other non-Manual	28	47	7	13
Farm	1	1	29	32
Other manual	35	11	34	13
Petty trading	10	5	13	6
n =	186	144	188	103

Any other classes?

It has been possible to identify the economic base for the formation of a middle class among young adults in the South Caucasus. Can we also identify other new or emergent classes? There are three candidates: a working class based on manual employment, a petit bourgeoisie (the self-employed), and an underclass (the unemployed and the inactive).

The obstacles to working-class formation extend beyond its ideological and cultural invisibility, as noted by previous commentators in Eastern Europe and the ex-USSR (see above). In the 1990s, during the economic downturns that followed the collapse of communism, the countries de-industrialized, and employment in their manufacturing industries has failed to recover. So in the South Caucasus few young adults had built stable careers in manual jobs– no more than 13 percent from any kind of family SES background were in our 'other employment' career group. Moreover, young people from all kinds of family backgrounds, and with and without higher education, were joining this career group in roughly equal proportions. Higher education being a prerequisite for a middle-class job did not mean that all higher-education graduates could expect such jobs (there were simply too many graduates). The potential working class was simply too small, its members' family SES and educational backgrounds were too diverse, and manual jobs were too unstable, to create a critical mass of family households with several members and intergenerational continuity in this potential class situation.

The self-employed were a relatively stable career group: 82 percent were still self-employed at the time of our survey. They had a higher continuity rate than any of the other employed, 16–30-age career groups. The main obstacles to class formation here were the diversity of their businesses, and self-employment tended to be a fall-back, a survival strategy, an alternative to chronic unemployment or inactivity, rather than a glamour career of choice. Among those who were self-employed at the time of the survey, 47 percent were farmers, typically on family farms. Another 18 percent were petty traders, buying and selling, usually on the streets. Others, a minority, were running construction, car repair, taxi businesses and suchlike. The earnings of the self-employed were generally inferior to those of employees in all kinds of jobs. A third said that their incomes were zero; they were usually working on family farms. Another two-fifths reported (adjusted) monthly earnings of less than \$100. Around a fifth of respondents without higher education from all kinds of family SES backgrounds had become self-employed. Whether or not respondents had been through higher education was the best guide to whether they would join this career group; only 1 in 20 university graduates had done so. The other useful predictor was gender: males were far more likely than females to be working on their own accounts.

Family farms were usually a household business with intergenerational continuity. Farm families could therefore be treated as an economic class. However, in most such households, farming was doing little more than enabling the residents to subsist. Rather than part of a petit bourgeoisie, we would portray such households, and most of those that were dependent on non-farm self-employment, as struggling to keep above an impoverished lower class. Meanwhile, a small minority of farm families had developed agriculture and animal husbandry into lucrative businesses, maybe combined with trading in farm produce from throughout their regions, thereby joining the middle class. Likewise, some urban businesses were generating incomes that gave households a middle-class lifestyle. Four percent of the self-employed had (adjusted) reported monthly earnings in excess of $500. Likewise, some manual jobs were well paid and stable, which, depending on the resources generated by other household members, could place these households at least within the periphery of their countries' middle classes.

Apart from the middle class, the only other cluster identifiable in our data with the characteristics of an economic class was a lower class comprising households whose adults were inactive, or chronically or intermittently unemployed. Many respondents were in these situations. Six percent of the males and 14 percent of the females were in the inactive career group. The males usually had 'conditions' – disabilities, injuries or chronic illnesses. The women were most likely to regard themselves as housewives. Another 24 percent of the males and 41 percent of the females were in the unemployment career group. This means that 30 percent of the males and 55 percent of the females had been mainly unemployed or inactive between age 16 and 30. Among those in the unemployed 16–30 career group, 58 percent had never held a proper job, and 62 percent were still unemployed at the time of our survey. Among those who had moved into jobs after age 30 (just 10 percent from the unemployment career group), roughly equal numbers had gained non-manual and other kinds of employment. Higher education was *not* reducing risks of entering the unemployed career group. It was family SES that had made a difference. Roughly two-fifths from the lowest SES band and one-fifth from the highest had become chronically unemployed. Many of those from the highest SES band were higher education graduates. After finishing university, they had evidently either preferred or been obliged to wait until they were able to start commensurate jobs. Maybe they knew that otherwise there was a danger of becoming typecast in non-graduate work, but this was a risky strategy because they ran the danger of being typecast as unemployable. However, unlike in the inactive career group, there was a significant volume of movement into and out of unemployment. At the same time, the sheer volume of unemployment and inactivity meant that there was a stratum of households with no one in regular, continuous work except, possibly, survival self-employment or subsistence-plus farming.

Social class

The aim here is not to test the existence of the economic classes identified above. We have shown that by 2007 middle and lower classes had been created as economic entities in the South Caucasus. The issue here is whether there were any corresponding social differences. If so, the social dimension would have been increasing the likelihood of the classes developing characteristic cultures, perpetuating themselves over time, and engaging in class-specific forms of political action, thereby making classes efficacious.

If the correct unit to classify is the family household rather than the individual, family behaviour is where we should expect some of the clearest indications of economic classes acquiring a social dimension, and we have data on the ages at which our respondents had made key family and housing life stage transitions. Table 10 gives the proportions who had married for the first time by age 23, and then by age 30. It shows that the non-manual career group was making the slowest progress in this respect. Individuals from this career group were the least likely to have married

Table 10. Career groups and family transitions (in percentages).

	Non-manual	Other employment	Self-employment	Unemployment	Inactive
Married by age 23	37	48	42	54	70
Not married at 23 but married by age 30	22	23	22	18	14
Unmarried at age 30	41	29	34	28	16
n =	290	134	166	391	118

at age 23, and were the most likely to be still single at 30. Conversely, our core, lower-class career groups, the unemployed and the inactive, were the most likely to be married at age 23, and the inactive group was the least likely to be still single at 30. The non-manual career group had reasons to delay marriage (while completing higher education and then establishing themselves in and progressing in employment careers) that simply did not apply in any of the other career groups.

Table 11 gives the percentages in the different career groups who resided with one or more parents (or parents-in-law) at age 25, and then at the time of the survey when the respondents were aged 31–37. Apart from the inactive (in the labour market) career group being the most likely to be living independently of family elders at both ages, there are no clear differences between the career groups, and over half from the inactive career group were still living with family elders at the time of the survey. We infer that the perpetuation of multi-generation living was classless in the South Caucasus, and that its persistence was more likely to be due to preference than to economic constraints. In the latter case, we would have expected the best-resourced, higher-income households, namely the middle-class households, to have enabled the highest proportion of their young married couples to live independently. This had not happened, and the highest earner among the 20 individuals who gave follow-up interviews (reported more fully below) – a male in Yerevan who was working for a Germany-based company – had actually bought two flats as an investment but, along with his wife and children, was continuing to live with his parents, and intended to maintain this arrangement as long as his parents lived. The relatively high proportion who had made housing transitions in the inactive career group could well have done so from exceptional constraints – the inability of the

Table 11. Career groups and housing transitions (in percentages).

	Non-manual	Other employment	Self-employment	Unemployment	Inactive
Living with parents (in-law) at age 25	85	88	87	83	75
Living with parents (in-law) at time of survey	72	76	70	69	58
n =	290	134	166	391	118

Table 12. Leisure profiles by labour market career groups.

	Non-manual	Other employment	Self-employment	Unemployment	Inactive
Percentages who never participated in three or more types of leisure activity	29	31	48	46	59
Percentages who maintained or increased at least two of 'going out', sport and high culture	20	13	7	6	13
Percentages who increased religious participation	20	17	16	17	11
Percentages who increased drinking and smoking	37	52	54	36	31
$n =$	290	134	166	391	118

young adults' families to accommodate all their male grown-up children, along with wives and younger children.

Our evidence on the young adults' uses of leisure has been reported fully elsewhere (see Roberts *et al.* 2009b). The key findings that are relevant here are summarized in Table 12. The 13 leisure activities on which respondents were questioned about their participation in each year from age 16 were reduced to five factors (groups of leisure activities which tended to be practised by the same individuals in the same year). The five leisure factors were going out (to the cinema, bars, etc.), high culture, sport, religion, and drinking and smoking. The top line in Table 12 gives the percentages in each of the labour market career groups who had never participated in three or more of these five types of leisure at any age. In other words, they had very low overall levels of leisure participation. This evidence shows that the employed career groups (the non-manuals and the other employment group, but not the self-employed) had the highest overall levels of leisure activity.

Participation in three out of the five kinds of leisure activity (going out, sport, and high culture) tended to have been maintained, risen or declined conjointly, and the second line in Table 12 shows that the non-manual career group had been the most likely to maintain or increase its involvement in these activities after age 16. They were mostly in the capital cities, where there were more opportunities to go to the cinema, restaurants, etc., than in the non-capital regions. Members of this middle-class group had the highest rates of involvement in these leisure activities to begin with, at age 16, and the difference between their level of involvement and the levels in other career groups widened with age. This widening is likely to have been associated with the greater likelihood of the non-manual group remaining single through their twenties and sometimes into their thirties.

Religious participation (attending services) had been the exception at all ages in all the career groups, though it was most common among the non-manuals and least common among the inactive (in the labour market) career group.

The only kinds of leisure activity and spending that rose overall after age 16 were drinking and smoking, and here the steepest rises were in the 'other employment' and 'self-employment' career groups. In most cases, their drinking and smoking was not in bars, restaurants and suchlike but in and around the young adults' homes. Most leisure time was spent 'hanging about', doing nothing in particular, or – the big time filler – watching television. Sustained involvement in any kind of formal, out-of-home leisure was far from universal within, but it was extremely rare outside, the middle-class group in the capital cities.

We conclude from this evidence that there are some clear indications of economic classes acquiring an additional social dimension.

Subjective class

We conducted a small number of follow-up interviews with selected respondents from the main survey, 20 in total across all three countries. There were equal numbers of males and females, and in the capital cities (where all the interviewees were higher-education graduates), and in the regions (where they were all from villages rather than the main towns). The questions included whether there were classes in the countries, and in which classes the respondents would place themselves. One person could not understand the questions. Another said that, 'There are no classes. There were in the 1990s but today everyone lives more or less the same.' The other 18 respondents answered without difficulty and usually without hesitation in describing their countries' classes.

There was agreement among these respondents on several points. First, everyone answered in terms of money. Second, they were all classifying their family households rather than just themselves. They spoke in terms of 'we' rather than 'I'. Third, everyone identified 'the rich' and sometimes added descriptors such as criminals, clans, and politicians. Just one interviewee placed his household 'maybe in the lower rich class': he was an exceptionally successful farmer.

Thereafter some used a two-class model, rich and poor (described as lowest by one respondent). They always placed themselves in the lowest or poor class. When respondents placed themselves among the poor, they were always placing themselves among the vast majority. None of these respondents fell into the middle class on our own definition.

The most popular class model was rich–middle–poor. Those who answered in these terms were divided on whether the middle class was the smallest, growing, or now the largest. With one exception, who placed his family 'between the poor and the middle class', those using the three-class model placed themselves in the middle class. Everyone who fell into the middle class on our definition self-described in this way, as did some who did not fall into our middle class on economic or social criteria.

No one mentioned the terms 'working class', 'underclass' or 'excluded groups'.

From this, we tentatively conclude – tentatively because of the small numbers – that the middle class had become the sole class of aspiration in the South Caucasus. In this sense, it really was the new 'holy' class (Ilyin 1998), having replaced communism's 'holy working class'. The rich were invariably (except by the sole 'lower rich' respondent) not envied but rather subjected to moral condemnation. Respondents were satisfied, often proud of their achievements, if they felt part of the middle class. They saw no prospect, and were not trying to join the rich. The poor were pitied rather than condemned. Above all else, to be middle class meant not to be poor.

Discussion and conclusions

We have argued that just two new classes have been formed in the post-communist South Caucasus (and probably in many other ex-communist territories). There is a new middle class with non-manual employees at its core, and a lower class with the chronically unemployed and economically inactive as its core members. These economic classes broadly correspond with the views of respondents who identified middle and poor classes, and we concede the existence of a rich, upper, capitalist class that was not captured in our fieldwork. We have also identified corresponding social differences, specifically in leisure and family careers. As expected, the same main classes were being formed in all the research locations. Azerbaijan was not exceptional. Earnings were rather higher, but not much higher, in Baku than in Tbilisi and Yerevan. So what was happening to the oil and gas revenues? Azerbaijan had more public building programmes (including the construction of a set of Olympic-grade sports facilities) than either Armenia or Georgia. Otherwise we suspect that the rich class in Azerbaijan had become richer than in the other South Caucasus countries.

The new classes in the South Caucasus are unlike the classes in the more mature, longer-established market economies of the West. There are several key differences, namely, that in the South Caucasus:

- All non-manual occupations fall within the middle classes.
- The family household is the unit that has to be classed.
- Manual occupations are insufficiently numerous and are too unstable to form the base for a working class.
- Small businesses are too varied, and too many of their proprietors are practising survival self-employment, to form a petit bourgeoisie.

A further difference, in our view, is that in the South Caucasus socio-economic classes are less likely to prove efficacious than were their Western counterparts during the twentieth century. There are several reasons for this.

First, one of the new classes is distinguished by its lack of employment, thus excluding the possibility of mobilization in occupation-based movements (trade unions and professional associations).

Second, up to now there has been no space for class-based politics in the South Caucasus. In Azerbaijan since 1993, all opposition to the incumbent regime has been suppressed, but even in Armenia and Georgia where elections are fiercely contested, the parties' agendas and the electoral contests have been dominated by non-class issues. The two issues that are likely to topple governments in the South Caucasus are territory (holding or regaining it) and corruption, and neither issue divides the populations on class lines.

Finally, in the South Caucasus, and so far everywhere else in the ex-communist realm, the sole inspiring vision of a better future is a version of the Western way of life. Young people may or may not be interested in long-term migration to the West. Their preference is usually for the Western way of life to spread into their own countries. Maybe at some point in the twenty-first century political movements will be created with alternative visions and programmes. Restoring the past – returning to Soviet-type socialism – is unlikely to appeal. Currently, there is a vacuum. The Western way of life has no serious competitor, yet we know that it is impossible for this way of life to spread to all the people on the planet.

Acknowledgements

The research reported in this paper was funded by INTAS, project 05-1000008-7803.

References

Abbott, P., 1987. Women's social class identification: does husband's occupation make a difference? *Sociology*, 21, 91–103.

Blanden, J., Gregg, P., and Machin, S., 2005. *Intergenerational mobility in Europe and North America*. London: Center for Economic Performance, London School of Economics.

Blossfeld, H.-P. and Timm, A., eds., 2003. *Who marries whom? Educational systems and marriage markets in modern societies*. Dordrecht: Kluwer.

Bogomolova, T., 1998. Income mobility in Russia in the mid-1990s. Paper presented at International Sociological Association Congress, Montreal.

Bridger, S., Kay, R., and Pinnick, K., 1996. *No more heroines? Russia, women and the market*. London: Routledge.

Britten, N. and Heath, A., 1983. Women, men and class analysis. *In*: E. Garmarnikow, D. Morgan, J. Purvis and D. Taylorson, eds. *Gender, class and work*. London: Heinemann.

Caucasus Research Resource Centre, 2005. *Data Initiative Survey 2005*, Baku/Tbilisi/Yerevan.

Charles, N., 1990. Women and class: a problematic relationship. *Sociological review*, 38, 43–89.

Erikson, R. and Goldthorpe, J.H., 1988. Women at class crossroads: a critical note. *Sociology*, 22, 545–553.

Evans, G. and Mills, C., 1999. Are there classes in post-communist societies? *Sociology*, 33, 23–46.

Eyal, G., Szelenyi, I., and Townsley, E., 1998. *Making capitalism without capitalists: the new ruling elites in Eastern Europe*. New York: Verso Books.

Goldthorpe, J.H., 1983. Women and class analysis. *Sociology*, 17, 465–488.

Hoffman, D.F., 2002. *The oligarchs: wealth and power in the new Russia*. Oxford: Public Affairs Limited.

Ilyin, V., 1998. The new middle strata in modern Russia. *In*: M. Kivinen, ed. *The Kalamari Union: middle class in East and West*. Aldershot: Ashgate, 118–129.

Khmelko, V., 2002. Macrosocial change in Ukraine: the years of independence. *Sisyphus*, 16, 125–135.

Kutsenko, O., 2002. Dynamics of class formation process in Ukrainian society. *Sisyphus*, 16, 137–150.

Leiulfsrud, H. and Woodward, A., 1987. Women at class crossroads: repudiating conventional theories of family class. *Sociology*, 21, 393–412.

Oksamytna, S. and Khemlko, V., 2004. Social exclusion in Ukraine in the initial stages of the restoring capitalism. *Ukrainian sociological review*, 4, 179–192.

Piirainen, T., 1998. From status to class: the emergence of a class society in Russia. *In*: M. Kivinen, ed. *The Kalamari Union: middle class in East and West*. Aldershot: Ashgate, 314–341.

Predborska, I., 2005. The social position of young women in present-day Ukraine. *Journal of youth studies*, 8, 349–365.

Roberts, K., 2005. Emergent class divisions among young adults in the former Soviet Union. *International Scope Review*, 7, 12 [online]. Available from: www.socialcapital-foundation, org/journal1/volume_2005/issue12/roberts.htm [Accessed 9 July 2009].
Roberts, K., Pollock, G., Manasyan, H., and Tholen, J., 2008. School-to-work transitions after two decades of post-communism: what's new?' *Eurasian journal of business and economics*, 1, 103–129.
Roberts, K., Pollock, G., Rustamova, S., Mammadova, Z., and Tholen, J., 2009a. Young adults' family and housing life-stage transitions during post-communist transitions in the South Caucasus. *Journal of youth studies*, 12, 151–166.
Roberts, K., Pollock, G., Tholen, J., and Tarkhnishvili L., 2009b. Youth leisure careers during post-communist transitions in the South Caucasus. *Leisure studies*, forthcoming.
Simonchuk, E., 2004. The working class in Ukraine: chronicle of losses. *Ukrainian sociological review*, 5, 155–178.
Stanworth, M., 1984. Women at class crossroads: a reply to Goldthorpe. *Sociology*, 18, 159–170.
Stenning, A., 2005. Where is the post-socialist working class? Working class lives in the spaces of (post)-socialism. *Sociology*, 39, 983–999.
Tilkidjiev, N., 1996. Social stratification in post-communist Bulgaria. *In*: J. Coen-Huther, ed., *Bulgaria at the crossroads.* New York: Nova Science Publishers, 79–96.
Tomanovic, S. and Ignjatovic, S., 2006. The transition of young people in a transition society: the case of Serbia. *Journal of youth studies*, 9, 269–285.
Trapido, D., 2007. Gendered transition: post-Soviet trends in gender wage inequality among young and full-time workers. *European sociological review*, 23, 223–237.
Wallace, C., 2002. Household strategies: their conceptual relevance and analytical scope in social research. *Sociology*, 36, 275–292.

Index

Page numbers in **Bold** represent figures.

Adams, M.: and Raisborough, J. 17-18
Addison, M.: and Taylor, Y. 7, 106
Ainley, P.: and Cohen, P. 59
Aldridge, J.: *et al* 30
anti-social behaviour orders (ASBO) 47
Arnett, J.J. 3

Ball, S.: *et al* 38
Barth, F. 11
Bauman, Z. 83; movement 104
Beck, U. 74, 77, 84, 105
Becker, H. 5, 33
Bennett, B.: and Tyler, I. 16
black, Asian and minority ethnic (BAME) people 59-61
black young men 6
Blackman, S.: youth studies 29
Blair, T. 27
Blossfeld, H.-P.: and Timm, A. 126
Bourdieu, P. 16, 22, 82, 85; habitus 70, 105
Bourgois, P. 68
Bradley, H. 59, 67
Brannen, J.: and Nilsen, A. 74
British economy 90
British gangs 26-7
British Sociological Association Youth Study Group 1
Bullock, K.: and Tilley, N. 28
Bynner, J. 3

capitalism 2-4
Cartmel, F.: and Furlong, A. 1, 6
Castell, S.: and Thompson, J. 3
Castells, M. 2
charvers *see* chavs
Chatterton, P.: and Hollands, R. 48-9, 104
chavs 4, 10, 14-16, 19, 116; appearance 16-17; behaviour 17; education 18-19; identity 22; talk 12
child poverty 3
class: economic 119; inequality 11-12; place 1, 39; post-communism 120; social 13, 119, 130; working 104, 107
Cohen, P. 75, 83; and Ainley, P. 59; reproduction codes 76
Cohen, S. 27; and Young, J. 47
Coles, B. 96
college studies 66-7
Colls, R.: and Lancaster, B. 104
Comedia 48
construction workforce: London 64
contemporary culture 56
contemporary post-industrial workplace 68
Criminal Justice and Public Order Act (1994) 28
Crouch, D. 48, 51
Cullen, G. 89, 99-100
cultural trends 1

de Certeau, M. 88
deindustrialization 76
Denzin, N. 97
detraditionalization 74
displacement 104
drug use: illegal 44-7, 52

East London 58
Ebbw Vale (Wales) 89-91; biographies 88; Blaenau Gwent 90; community regeneration 96; continuity 89, 100;

discontinuity 99, 101; former steelworks site **90**, 93-5; industrial transformation 100-1; land use plan **98**; life-course passage 95; master plan 90, 98, **99**; post-industrial transformation 91; sociology of youth transitions 92; step-change 93-4; topographical 90; transitions into adulthood 88
economic classes 119
education 10, 18-19
emergent class formations 119
ethnicity subculture 14
Evans, K.: *et al* 82
excessive corporeality 16

femininity: traditional 110
feminized labour force 103; new femininities 105
Furlong, A.: and Cartmel, F. 1, 6

gang areas 26
non-gang involved 26, 30
gangs 15; affected neighbourhood 38-9; British 26-7; Eurogang definition 30; exclusion from school 37; gun crime 28, 31; labels 32-4, 36; Las Vegas 28; low aspirations 37; members 33-4; police harassment tactic 35-6; policing 28, 33-4; USA 28; victimization 31-2; YOGEC (youth gangs in an English city) ethnographic study 30
Giddens, A. 77, 97, 105
graffiti 51
grafting 6, 58, 64-6; grafter culture 69
Griffin, C.: and Holt, M. 16
Guardian 27
gun crime: gangs 28, 31
Gunter, A.: and Watt, P. 5-7

Hagedorn, J. 29
Hall, T.: *et al* 6-7, 92-3
Hallsworth, S.: and Young, T. 27
Hamnett, C. 61
Hampson, T. 4
Harvey, D. 2, 48
Henderson, S.: *et al* 97
hippies 13
Hobbs, D. 60
Holland, J.: and Thomson, R. 74
Hollands, R.: and Chatterton, P. 48-9, 104
Hollingworth, S. 4; and Williams, K. 12
Holt, M.: and Griffin, C. 16
Home Office: Tackling Gangs Action Programme (TGAP) 27
Hood, R.: and Joyce, K. 60

Ignjatović, S.: and Tomanović, S. 74
Ilyin, V. 121, 133
individualization 3; Russia (post-Soviet) 74, 83
Ingold, T. 89, 97-9, 101
interpretative repertoires 16

Jameson, F. 2, 4
Johnston, L.: *et al* 64
Journal of Youth Studies 3

Katz, C.: and Webb, V. 28
Kehily, M.J.: and Nayak, A. 105
Khmelko, V. 120
Kintrea, K.: *et al* 29-30, 40
Klee, P. 97
Klein, M. 29
Kutsenko, O. 120

Lancaster, B.: and Colls, R. 104
Lawler, S. 116; class inequality 11-12
Lefebvre, H. 48
leisure 5; practices 51-2; spaces 44-5, 56
Lemert, E. 33
liminality 54
Lloyd, T. 65
Loader, I. 53
London 60; Canary Wharf 60; construction workforce 64, 69; East 60; poorest neighbourhoods 61; socio-spatial polarization 61; working class 14
Lucey, H.: and Reay, D. 83

McAra, L.: and McVie, S. 34
McCorkle, R.: and Miethe, T. 28
McCulloch, K.: *et al* 10, 13
MacDonald, R.: *et al* 29, 39, 58, 67, 69; and Marsh, J. 52, 54, 74, 76; and Shildrick, T. 10, 29, 59-60

McVie, S.: and McAra, L. 34
Marsh, J.: and MacDonald, R. 52, 54, 74, 76
Marshall, M.: *et al* 40
Marx, K. 2
Meadows, P. 65
methodological approaches 7
Miethe, T.: and McCorkle, R. 28
Morgan, R. 27

Nayak, A. 10, 110, 116; chav 20; and Kehily, M.J. 105; social class 13; working class 104
neighbourhood: East London 58, 62; gang-affected 39; inner-city 40; London's poorest 61
nightscapes 44, 48-9; nightclubs 49
Nilsen, A.: and Brannen, J. 74
normative selfhood 11, 18
North-East England 103; Bigg Market 110-11; branded identity crisis 114; Bridge Burn 114; changing landscapes 106; class analysis 106; de-industrialization 117; degeneration 107; displacement 104; economic transformation 107; gender and class 116; Jasmine Vale 114; leisure space 111-12; Millfield 115; mining 109; public sociology 108; Quayside 112; racism 116; real Geordie identity 104, 110; rejuvenation via leisure 110; traditional femininity 110; transition 106; urban mobility 109, 116; urban transformation 113, 116; working class 107; young working class women (accounts) 111; younger women 104

occupation 119
Organization for Economic Co-operation and Development (OECD) 91
othering 11

People United Against Crime 53
Piirainen, T. 120
place: class 1, 39
play work 67
police harassment tactic: gangs 35-6
Pollock, G.: and Roberts, K. 7, 121, 123
poshies 13
post-communism: class 120
post-subcultural studies 10
Potter, J.: and Wetherell, M. 16
pregnancy 54
The Punitive City (Cohen) 38

racial discrimination 70
Raisborough, J.: and Adams, M. 17-18
Ralphs, R.: *et al* 5, 7
Reay, D.: and Lucey, H. 83
Reynolds, T. 63
Rich, A. 4
road culture 62-4; badness 67-8
Roberts, K.: and Pollock, G. 7, 121, 123
Robinson, C. 5, 46
Russia (post-Soviet) 73, 86; active role by parents 81-2; compulsory education 78-9; degradation of opportunities 82; higher education 83-4; individualization 74, 83; industrial and agricultural sectors 74; informal networks 75; inheritance 82-3; initial vocational education and training (IVET) system 74-5, 77-8; peer influence 81; state-led economic system 73-4; training courses gendered nature 81; transitions to adulthood 75; Ulyanovsk 74, 77, 85
Russian economy early 1990s 77

Savage, M.: *et al* 105
Sayer, A. 15-16
school: Urban state 12
school exclusion 64
schooling: social class 10
Sennett, R. 81
serial vision 99-100
Shildrick, T.: and MacDonald, R. 10, 29, 59-60
Skeggs, B. 11, 16, 17, 113; class 13, 22; subject of value 18
social class 2, 10, 119, 130; identities 4; schooling 10
social exclusion 38
social policies 3
social scientific study of youth 1

social theorists 29
socio-spatial marginality 59
South Caucasus study: Armenia 121, 126, 134; Azerbaijan 121, 126, 134; career groups 122; current occupations **123**; family farms 129; family household 128; family socio-economic status 126; family transitions **131**; gender 123-4; Georgia 121, 126, 134; higher education investment 126, **128**; households 122; housing transitions **131**; jobs **128**; labour market **122, 123, 124**; leisure profiles 132, **132**; lower class 130; marriage 130-1; multi-generation living 125, 131; new middle class 126, 133; non-manual employment 128; parental data **127**; personal incomes **124**; religious participation 133; sectors of employment **125**; self-employment 129; social class 130; subjective class 133; western way of life 135; women in public sector employment 125; working class formation 129
Southerton, D. 21
space 48; consumerized 48; free 44, 48, 56; leisure 44-5, 56; memory 50; public 53
storytelling 56
Strangleman, T. 85
street 51
studies: post-subcultural 10
subculture 12-14, 19; ethnicity 14
The Sun 27

Tackling Gangs Action Programme (TGAP): Home Office 27
Taylor, Y.: and Addison, M. 7, 106
Thompson, J.: and Castell, S. 3
Thomson, R.: and Holland, J. 74
Thorne, B.: border work 11
Thrift, N. 89, 101; urban catastrophe 94
Tilley, N.: and Bullock, K. 28
Timm, A.: and Blossfeld, H.-P. 126
Tita, G.: *et al* 29, 32, 36
Tkach, O. 77
Tomanović, S.: and Ignjatović, S. 74
transition: school-to-work 65, 69; young males 58; youth 1, 54-5, 59
transport: wayfarer 97-8
Turner, V. 54; liminoid 55
Tyler, I. 4; and Bennett, B. 16; chav celebrities 19; class 13

University of Teesside 59
urban state schools 12

Van Gennep, A. 54
Venkatesh, S.A. 29
Vigil, J.D. 29

Wacquant, L. 59
Wales 88
Walker, C. 6, 74, 84
Walkerdine, V.: *et al* 95
Watt, P. 69; and Gunther, A. 5-7
wayfarer: transport 97-8
Webb, V.: and Katz, C. 28
Welsh Assembly Government 90
Western-sourced class schemes 120
Wetherell, M.: and Potter, J. 16
white middle class 14-15
Williams, K.: and Hollingworth, S. 12
Williams, R. 81
Willis, P.: school-to-work transition 65; street 51; working-class masculinity 18, 82
women 7, 103; white middle-class 106; white working-class 106
Woodman, D. 3
working class 104; identity 76; London 14; North East England 107; routes to adulthood 73
working-class masculinity 18, 104

Young, J.: and Cohen, S. 47
Young, T.: and Hallsworth, S. 27
youth: transition 1, 54-5, 59
youth culture 2
Youth Justice Board 27
youth studies: Teesside 92
youth work 67